FLIGHT/VIDAS

User Manual

Fort Lauderdale, Florida

Enalan Communications, Inc.

2015

FLIGHT/VIDAS User Manual

Enalan Communications, Inc., Fort Lauderdale
Florida.

First printing, October, 2015

CS edition

For the most up-to-date information on the FLIGHT/VIDAS project and to learn how to access assessment materials, go to:

www.flightvidas.org

Acknowledgments

The development of a new measure of health literacy required a coordinated team effort without which the project would not have been successful. The contributions of the FLIGHT/VIDAS team members are gratefully acknowledged:

Amarilis Acevedo, PhD
Drenna Waldrop-Valverde, PhD
Sara Czaja, PhD
David Loewenstein, PhD
Ana-Maria Homs, PsyD
Rosemary Davenport, RN, MSN, ARNP
Robin Jacobs, PhD
Joshua Caballero, PharmD
Lillian Valiente
Jamie Mazzurco, DO, MPH

The FLIGHT/VIDAS project was supported by grants from the National Heart Lung and Blood Institute (R01HL096578 and 2R56HL096578) to Dr. Ownby.

Contents

1 Introduction

Thanks to the pioneering work of early researchers and educators, over the past several decades health literacy has become prominent in discussions of health and health education. People who don't understand their health and don't know how to find out about it can have trouble getting the healthcare they need. Health literacy is key in helping people understand how to become and stay healthy, and those who have low levels of health literacy deserve to have communications about their health in a form and content they can understand.

Increasing attention to health literacy has highlighted a number of issues about what health literacy is and how it should be measured. Several helpful conceptual definitions of health literacy have been proposed, such as those Healthy People 2020 (Department of Health and Human Services, 2011), the definition in the 2004 Institute of Medicine report (Nielsen-Bohlman, Panzer, & Kindig, 2004) , and the Calgary Charter (The Centre for Health Literacy, 2011). In fact, one review article (Sorensen et al., 2013) found 17 definitions and 12 conceptual models of health literacy. While these definitions are useful, how they can be translated on the ground to create assessment tools and interventions to improve health literacy is not always clear. Statements such as "the ability to obtain and use health information" are a critical first step, but how, specifically, do we measure the "ability to obtain . . . health information?" Our efforts to identify, measure, and intervene with persons with low health literacy demand better assessment tools–tools that can efficiently identify individuals' health literacy needs, effectively address those needs, and measure the effects of those interventions.

Efforts to address issues related to low health literacy also demand better assessment tools. Even such broad solutions as the "universal precautions" approach, in which all information is presented at a level that most individuals can understand, require assessment of the target individuals' health literacy. Baseline level of health literacy is likely to be an important factor in how well people understand information presented, even when it has been made as understandable as possible. This kind of assessment of baseline health literacy would address an important question about the universal precautions approach: What about people whose health literacy is so low that even the materials created for universal precautions is still too difficult? Our research suggests that a substantial number of individuals may need information provided with auditory support such as narration and with carefully chosen graphics to support verbal information. In the FLIGHT/VIDAS project, we identified a small but significant subgroup of individuals who had very low levels of health literacy. We need to know how best to address their needs for health information, and without baseline assessment and evaluation of the effects of interventions, we simply won't know. All these efforts thus depend on the ability to operationally define and measure health literacy. If a person's level of health literacy cannot be reliably determined, research on the effects of health literacy on their health or the impact of an intervention on their health literacy cannot be done in a way that yields meaningful information.

Why another health literacy measure?

The limitations of measures of health literacy have been discussed elsewhere (Baker, 2006; Jordan, Osborne, & Buchbinder, 2011; Pleasant, McKinney, & Rikard, 2011). Previously available measures have been criticized for assessing a limited set of skills and for their development using patients drawn from single racial, ethnic, age, or socioeconomic groups.

Other criticisms have noted the limited content and face validity of the measures and lack of evidence on the measures' construct validity (Jordan et al., 2011). Further, although both Spanish and English versions of several measures are available, they were not developed using psychometric procedures that assure their equivalence. Because of this, it is not possible to make valid comparisons of health literacy across language groups.

From a research perspective, one of the most important problems with current health literacy measures is that each assesses a different aspect of health literacy, making it difficult to know whether studies that use different measures mean the same thing. From a clinical perspective, it's hard to know how to identify people with low health literacy, since the measures don't agree when used for this purpose (Haun, Luther, Dodd, & Donaldson, 2012; Ramirez-Zohfeld, 2015). Whether in clinical or research settings, most measures of health literacy must be administered, scored, and interpreted by trained clinicians, making them time and cost intensive.

Pleasant et al. (2011) argue that new measures of health literacy should be multidimensional and assess health literacy as a latent construct. A multidimensional approach would recognize that functional health literacy comprises a number of distinct skills or abilities, such as reading, listening, and performing quantitative operations (Nielsen-Bohlman et al., 2004). Evaluation of latent constructs is frequently used in psychological assessment to study an ability or trait that cannot be directly measured. Multiple test items believed to be related are administered and then what they have in common is statistically extracted, usually with factor analysis. Many item response theory models approach the measurement of abilities as latent constructs and have been used to develop assessments of health literacy. Pleasant et al. (2011) also suggest that assessments should recognize that measures are most likely to be accurate when they are similar to the context in which the actual behavior occurs. Assessment using a video simulation of a clinical encounter, for example, may be more accurate than asking for responses to written questions. In F/V, we addressed these issues by ensuring we included diverse item contents and employing a psychometrically rigorous latent variable modeling approach in evaluating the new measure's construct validity. We also included video simulations of health care encounters to make our assessments as similar to real-life situations as possible (see Chapter 3 for details).

An issue limiting the usefulness of several measures is their response format. The TOFHLA, for example, uses the cloze procedure (Ackerman, Beier, & Bowen, 2000) to assess reading comprehension. With this strategy, comprehension is tested by asking the person assessed to supply a word missing in a sentence (e.g., "The sky is _____"). The cloze procedure creates items that are differentially more difficult for older persons. Cloze performance is related to information processing speed and verbal fluency, reduced in older persons (Ackerman & Cianciolo, 2000), and data from two separate studies indicate that age-related differential item functioning exists on a significant number of items from the reading comprehension subtest of the TOFHLA (Ownby & Waldrop-Valverde, 2013; Ownby, Acevedo, Waldrop-Valverde, & Jacobs, 2014). In one of these studies (Ownby et al, 2014), eliminating the items that were biased against older persons actually eliminated age-group differences in overall scores. In F/V, we addressed this issue by creating items that allow users to choose one among several possible answers and evaluated items for age– and language–related differential item functioning.

As noted, almost all existing measures require hand scoring, making them time– and effort–intensive. Clearly, a computer–administered and scored measure of health literacy would make assessment more accessible in both clinical and research settings by reducing demands on clinician or researcher time while better standardizing the measure's administration. Integration of such a measure into an electronic health record might allow for inclusion of health literacy scores into patients' health records. This type of integration would allow for transmission of information about patients' level of health literacy directly to treating clinicians, allowing them to better understand their patients' information needs. The automated assessment of health literacy might also allow for the individualized tailoring of health–related information to level of health literacy, a strategy previously shown to be effective in influencing patient behavior (Noar, Benac, & Harris, 2007; Lustria et al., 2013;Ownby, Hertzog, & Czaja, 2012), and which may be effective in reducing health disparities (Jerant, Sohler, Fiscella, Franks, & Franks, 2011).

It was in this context when in 2005 we set out to develop a new measure of health literacy. We chose to create a measure with diverse health-related content that would be computer administered and scored. We wanted it to be acceptable to diverse groups and equivalent in both English and Spanish and among younger and older persons. The remainder of this manual describes the process by which we developed the new measure of health literacy and how we have worked to make it valid and useful to others. This measure of health literacy was developed in a way that addressed previous criticisms. It samples a wide range of content chosen from the health literacy domains proposed in the influential 2004 Institue of Medicine (IOM) report on health literacy (Nielsen-Bohlman et al., 2004). It is based on a coherent conceptual model of health literacy (outlined in Chapter 2) that has been developed based on our own and others' research. It includes items that assess prose, document, and quantitative literacies in each of the IOM domains. It was developed through a rigorous multi-stage process (see Chapter 3) in which items have been pilot tested, assessed for equivalence in both English and Spanish as well as in younger and older individuals, and subjected to assessments of construct, concurrent, and known groups validity.

It assesses not only reading and quantitative skills but also uses video simulations of healthcare related encounters to assess listening comprehension and to provide test stimuli that bear a close relation to the actual situations in which health literacy skills might be applied. By asking questions that assess expressive writing skills (by asking, for example, where certain kinds of information would be placed in a form) the measure indirectly assesses expressive written language skills. The new measure utilizes a broad range of item formats and contents, includes listening comprehension, and has been developed in English and Spanish. The English portion of our project is named ***Fostering Literacy for Good Health Today (FLIGHT)*** and the related Spanish project is V***ive Desarollando Amplia Salud (VIDAS)***. In the rest of this manual, we'll refer to the project as ***F/V.***

Overview

The purpose of this manual is give those interested in the assessment of health literacy the information needed to make informed decisions about how to use the scales developed in the FLIGHT/VIDAS project. Although we've published information about its development, reliability, and validity elsewhere (Ownby, Acevedo, Waldrop-Valverde, Jacobs, & Caballero, 2013; Ownby et al., 2013; Ownby, Acevedo, Waldrop-Valverde, Jacobs, & Caballero, 2014; Ownby, Acevedo, Jacobs, Caballero, & Waldrop-Valverde, 2014b; Ownby, Acevedo, Jacobs, Caballero, & Waldrop-Valverde, 2014a; Ownby et al., 2014; Ownby, Acevedo, Goodman, Caballero, & Waldrop-Valverde, 2015), we hope that this manual will bring all this information together in one place for more convenient access. In addition, since some of the publications referenced were based on interim data analyses, those presented here are based on the final dataset created at the end of the project. Appendixes I–III provide author manuscripts of several of these earlier peer-reviewed publications.

In addition, this manual presents data on two previously-unreported scales that have been created primarily in response to feedback from potential users. While our main focus in creating F/V was to develop a computer-administered and scored measure of health literacy that could be used to tailor computer-delivered interventions to improve health literacy, many potential F/V users made it clear to us that while computer administration would be helpful in many situations, many users still work in places where computers and Internet access would be complicated or simply not available. As explained in Chapter 3, Development, in initial item development we created more than 225 items, and in the final development phase we extensively tested 98 of them. A number of these items could be administered without a computer or Internet connection, and we were able to develop a 20-item scale that can be administered in a paper and pencil format. Further, in response to many questions about the use of F/V to quickly identify individuals who are likely to have limited health literacy skills, we created a 10-item screening scale that will require only a few minutes to administer and score. It can be used to quickly identify individuals likely to have low health literacy. Information on how to obtain the test booklet and answer sheets is available on the F/V website (www.flightvidas.org). Information on the reliability and validity of these scales is presented in Chapter 4.

The overall plan of this manual is first to explain in this introduction why we created F/V, then to go on and detail the conceptual model that underlies F/V in chapter 2, The ASK Model. Chapter 3 reviews in greater detail the steps taken to develop F/V items include preliminary psychometric assessments, while Chapter 4 provides more detail on the measure including final data on scale reliability and validity. Chapter 5 includes tables with T scores across language and age groups. These tables are reproduced in the final Appendix in order to make them easy to access when using F/V.

2 The ASK Model

Overview

Health literacy, defined as an individuals' ability to obtain and use health information to make choices about health care, is related in many way to their health (Berkman, Sheridan, Donahue, Halpern, & Crotty, 2011), health status, service utilization, self-care behaviors, and even risk for death (Baker, Wolf, Feinglass, & Thompson, 2008). It has also been tied to race– and ethnicity–related disparities (Osborn et al., 2011). Even with ongoing research, though, important questions about health literacy remain. One key question is how health literacy can be operationally defined so it can be measured and interventions to improve it can be developed.

This problem arises from the diverse ways health literacy has been defined and the varying content and format of widely-used health literacy measures. For example, in most studies, health literacy has implicitly defined as a person's performance on a test of health literacy. Since each of the most commonly–used health literacy tests measures it in a different way, it is difficult to know exactly what these studies mean. In some cases, health literacy has been assessed as a person's ability to demonstrate that he or she understands health–related information. This strategy underlies the Reading subtest of Test of Functional Health Literacy in Adults, or TOFHLA (Parker, Baker, Williams, & Nurss, 1995). In other studies, health literacy is defined as a person's ability to correctly pronounce health–related words, as with the Rapid Estimate of Adult Literacy in Medicine, or REALM (Murphy, Davis, Long, Jackson, & Decker, 1993) or to identify synonyms of health-related words as in the Short Assessment of Health Literacy for Spanish Adults, or SAHLSA (Lee, Bender, Ruiz, & Cho, 2006). Each of these strategies assesses something related to health literacy, but their diversity leaves open the question of what each has in common with the "social construct of health literacy" (Pleasant, McKinney, & Rikard, 2011).

Each measure samples different content, uses different response formats, and has been developed on different populations (Haun, Luther, Dodd, & Donaldson, 2012). The TOFHLA, for example, evaluates reading comprehension by asking a person to supply words eliminated from the text (the cloze procedure), while its numeracy scale asks that he or she explain how to take medications. The REALM requires the person to correctly read aloud words related to healthcare. The need for a similar measure for Spanish speakers led to the development of the SAHLSA, but the low frequency of orthographically-irregular words in Spanish meant that it was necessary to develop a different response format. The SAHLSA asks the person tested to view a stimulus word on a card and choose which of two other words is most similar in meaning.

Performance on these measures requires basic reading skills and conceptual health knowledge, and several, especially the TOFHLA subtests, also require reasoning, problem solving and numeracy skills (Ownby & Waldrop-Valverde, 2009). The variety of contents and formats, however, suggests that the abilities required for successful performance on each are different (Haun et al., 2012; Jordan, Osborne, & Buchbinder, 2011). Griffin et al., for example, showed substantial differences in which patients were identified as having limited health literacy by different measures (Griffin et al., 2010), and similar findings have been reported in other studies (Haun et al., 2012; Osborn et al., 2007).

Because of these issues, in developing F/V we hypothesized that more clearly establishing the relations of health literacy measures to other factors might provide a better understanding of what each measures. We also hypothesized that a better understanding would also provide a clearer picture of health literacy by defining its component skills. In the study we review in this chapter, based on reviews of empirical research and conceptual models of health literacy, we hypothesized that after taking into account individuals' social and cultural contexts, the variables most relevant to health literacy would be their general cognitive abilities, academic skills, and health-related knowledge.

Health Literacy's Social Context

Studies have shown that health literacy is related to age, race, ethnicity, and socioeconomic status. For example, persons older than 65 years of age performed at lower levels on the Health Literacy scale of the National Assessment of Adult Literacy (Kutner, Greenberg, Jin, & Paulsen, 2006). Blacks and Hispanics have also been shown to perform at lower levels on measures of health literacy. Closely intertwined with other demographic characteristics is socioeconomic status, itself related to health literacy (Paasche-Orlow & Wolf, 2007). The finding that English-speaking Hispanics may be at a disadvantage to non-Hispanics when their health literacy is assessed in English (Aguirre, Ebrahim, & Shea, 2005) suggests that preferred language may also be a key characteristic. Gender has also been related to performance on tests of health literacy (Aguirre et al., 2005). For purposes of measuring the broader context in which individuals exist, in F/V we assessed sociocultural factors such as race, ethnicity, gender, acculturation, education, income, and occupational status. These were taken into account in data analyses in order to place our participants' health literacy in an appropriate social context.

Cognitive Abilities

Understanding the relation of tests of health literacy to basic cognitive abilities (or general intellectual abilities, often assessed by IQ tests) may be especially important since research has shown that both general intellectual abilities and health literacy are related to health (Baker et al., 2002; Chin et al., 2011; Mottus et al., 2014; Wolf et al., 2012). General intellectual ability can be defined as reflecting a person's acquired knowledge and communication ability, crystallized ability, and capacity to reason and solve novel problems, often referred to as fluid ability (Horn & Cattell, 1966). Baker et al. (2002) showed that overall performance on the Mini-mental State Exam (Folstein, Folstein, & McHugh, 1975) was related to S-TOFHLA scores. Levinthal et al. (2008) evaluated the relation of demographic and cognitive variables to performance on the S-TOFHLA. Chin et al. (2011) found that age, education, basic cognitive abilities, and disease-related knowledge were all related to performance on the S-TOHLA and REALM. Others have shown that performance on tests of health literacy is related to various cognitive abilities including memory, verbal fluency, reasoning, and general intellectual functioning (Federman, Sano, Wolf, Siu, & Halm, 2009; Wolf et al., 2012; Yost, Dewalt, Lindquist, & Hahn, 2013).

Academic Skills

By its very nature, health literacy is related to academic skills such as reading and mathematics (Baker, 2006). Academic skills can be distinguished from basic cognitive abilities by their acquisition via formal instruction during schooling. While basic cognitive abilities are thought to be stable over time (Deary, Pattie, & Starr, 2013), academic skills such as reading, writing, and arithmetic are amenable to change through formal interventions well into adult life (Kruidenier, MacArthur, & Wrigley, 2010). While it is important to distinguish between general reading skills and health literacy (Nielsen-Bohlman, Panzer, & Kindig, 2004), the correlation between patients' performance on measures of academic skills and health literacy has also been used to validate health literacy measures (Bass, III, Wilson, & Griffith, 2003; Parker et al., 1995).

Conceptual Health Knowledge

In addition to social context, cognitive abilities and academic skills, health knowledge is related both to performance on tests of health literacy and health. Disease-specific knowledge, for example, has been linked to health literacy in diabetes (Rothman et al., 2005), hypertension (Chin et al., 2011; Gazmararian, Williams, Peel, & Baker, 2003), HIV infection (Hicks,

Barragan, Franco-Paredes, Williams, & Del, 2006), asthma, and congestive heart failure (Gazmararian et al., 2003). This makes sense, since even persons with excellent reading skills may have difficulty understanding material based on unfamiliar concepts. Again, conceptual health knowledge can be differentiated from basic cognitive abilities because it clearly can be taught. It is also different from academic skills as it only requires a person to demonstrate understanding of specific facts rather than more complex sequences of behaviors required for skills.

Health Literacy as Expertise

Several authors have noted the close relation of performance on measures of health literacy to general cognitive ability and concluded that the individual differences in health literacy may primarily reflect underlying differences general cognitive ability (Mottus et al., 2014; Wolf et al., 2012). In our approach to developing a measure of health literacy, we believed it was important to take many factors related to health and health literacy into account as we developed an operational model of health literacy that could inform assessment and intervention. We believe, however, that the conclusion that measures of health literacy are related to health only or primarily because of their underlying relation to general cognitive ability is overly simplistic and neglects important factors related to health literacy that can affect health and health disparities. Further, this interpretation has important implications for policy in developing interventions to improve health literacy. Reducing health literacy to individual differences in general cognitive abilities could lead to a nihilistic attitude about efforts to improve health literacy. If general cognitive ability is key, and it is difficult or impossible to change, what is the point of trying to improve health literacy?

For F/V, we developed an alternative model of health literacy based on an analysis of health literacy performances as a form of expertise. Expert performance has been studied in a number of domains, ranging from playing chess to sight reading music (Charness & Tuffiash, 2008). This approach is apt because, like other forms of expertise, understanding and applying health information to make healthcare choices requires a combination of general intellectual abilities, specific skills, and task-related knowledge. For example, while general cognitive ability is important in becoming proficient at chess, the specific ability of visual working memory may be particularly important (Reingold, Charness, Pomplun, & Stampe, 2001). Still, a high IQ and good visual working memory do not make a chess master—skilled performance in playing chess requires knowledge of rules and the capacity to recognize sequences of moves that constitute recognizable patterns that come only with learning and practice (Roring & Charness, 2007). In a similar way, obtaining, understanding, and using health information requires basic cognitive abilities, academic skills in reading and numeracy, and conceptual knowledge related to specific issues such as disease pathophysiology and treatment or health promotion through diet and exercise. From this point of view, differences in cognitive ability, socioeconomic status, education, reading ability and many other factors are all important. This analysis has important policy implications as well and avoids the nihilism of reducing health literacy to general cognitive ability and provides direction for developing interventions to address differences in health literacy. While it may be difficult to change a person's general cognitive ability, it is clearly possible to improve reading and math skills as well as to teach health–related knowledge.

The ASK Model

The studies reviewed above illustrate the core abilities and skills related to health literacy and that conceptual knowledge as well is a key factor. Basic cognitive abilities, academic skills, and health knowledge are each related to performance on measures of health literacy. Few studies of health literacy, however, have included measures assessing all of these domains. Further, studies that have used variables from multiple domains have shown that variables from one domain may affect the importance of others, as when inclusion of a measure of general intellectual ability reduc-

Table 2-1. Final regression analysis for ASK model

	B	SE	Beta	*t*	*p*
Intercept	7.51	2.35	n/a	3.20	0.001
Language	-1.58	0.40	-0.14	-3.96	< 0.001
Gender	0.06	0.33	0.01	0.18	0.86
Race	-0.95	0.43	-0.08	-2.22	0.03
Age	-0.14	0.01	-0.45	-15.86	< 0.001
SES[a]	0.67	0.18	0.12	3.74	< 0.001
Social Status[a]	-0.07	0.08	-0.02	-0.88	0.38
Crystallized[a]	0.10	0.02	0.21	5.12	< 0.001
Fluid[a]	0.00	0.00	0.01	0.37	0.71
Reading[a]	0.09	0.02	0.18	4.44	< 0.001
Knowledge[a]	0.68	0.07	0.34	9.80	< 0.001

[a]SES = socioeconomic status index derived from principal components analysis of education, income, and occupational status; Social Status= Participant self rating on McArthur Foundation subjective social status ladder; Crystallized = crystallized intellectual ability; Fluid = fluid intellectual ability; Reading = Woodcock-Johnson or Woodcock-Muñoz Passage Comprhension subtest; Knowledge = F/V conceptual health knowledge scale.

es the importance of other factors in health. In creating F/V, we hypothesized that understanding health literacy as the property of an individual required taking into account a person's social context, as emphasized by many authors. This aspect of individuals' health literacy was assessed as their age, gender, race, and socioeconomic status (a composite of educa-

Table 2-2. Variability in health literacy related to social context, cognitive ability, reading, and knowledge

Model	R	R^2	Adj R^2	SE	Δ^a	*p*
1[b]	0.66	0.43	0.43	4.28	0.43	<.001
2[b]	0.76	0.58	0.57	3.70	0.15	<.001
3[b]	0.78	0.60	0.60	3.58	0.03	<.001
4[b]	0.82	0.67	0.67	3.26	0.07	<.001

[a]Δ = change in R^2 value related to each group of variables in Models 1 to 4.
[b]Model 1 = social context variables only; Model 2 adds crystallized and fluid general ability; Model 3 adds reading comprehension; Model 4 adds conceptual health knowledge.

tion, income, and occupational status).

Given the body of research showing the importance of general intellectual abilities in health literacy and health outcomes, participants in F/V completed a brief battery of cognitive measures that allowed us to take crystallized and fluid intellectual ability into account in understanding their health literacy. We also recognized, as do others, that academic skills are important in understanding health literacy. In order to take this into account, participants in F/V completed a standardized measure of academic skills that was developed in both English and Spanish, either the Woodcock-Johnson (English) or Woodcock-Muñoz (Spanish) reading comprehension and applied mathematics problems subtests (Woodcock, McGrew, & Mather, 2007; Woodcock, Muñoz-Sandoval, McGrew, & Mather, 2007).

Finally, based on our analysis of health literacy as a form of expertise, we believed that conceptual health knowledge (knowledge of specific facts about disease and health) would be important aspects of health literacy. While there are a number of disease-specific knowledge measures, no general health knowledge measure that was both brief and validated was readily available. As part of creating F/V we therefore included a number of conceptual health knowledge questions. We hypothesized that, as with general information as assessed in the Wechsler intelligences scales (Wechsler, 1944; Wechsler, 1958), it might be possible to identify a group of health-related factual questions that, when included in a scale of 10 to 15 items, would be a useful measure of general health knowledge. As is further discussed in Chapters 3 and 4, we were successful in creating such a scale.

The final conceptual model thus specified that after taking social context into account, the key factors that define an individual's health literacy are basic cognitive abilities, core academic skills, and health-related knowledge (ASK). In a published study, we examined how well this model predicted our participants' performance on the measures of health literacy included in our assessment battery. All participants completed either the English or Spanish version of the TOFHLA, with English-speaking participants completing the REALM and Spanish-speaking participants completing the SAHLSA. Participants also completed the final 98-item set of F/V questions.

By examining the relation of these groups of variables to our participants' scores on each measure, we sought to evaluate the contribution of each group to health literacy. Results of the final statistical model for F/V are presented in Table 2-1. The contribution of each group to each measure as R-squared values is presented in Table 2-2.

Summary

Our data thus clearly support the ASK model. Rather than reducing health literacy to general cognitive ability, the model supports the complexity of an individual's health literacy embedded in social context, educational background, and learning experiences as well as ability. It should be noted that although we have only presented an analysis of the ASK model for F/V, in the past we published data on its applicability to other measures of health literacy (Ownby, Acevedo, Waldrop-Valverde, Jacobs, & Caballero, 2014). These data in general support the model's wider relevance to other measures of health literacy. A copy of the manuscript for this paper, with information on the ASK model and the TOFHLA, REALM, and SAHLSA, is included in this manual as Appendix III (page 149).

3 Development

Overview

The measure that has become FLIGHT/VIDAS went through an extensive development process that began in 2005 with pilot testing of health literacy items on an early consumer-oriented touch screen computer in a clinic at the University of Miami. Subsequently, with support from the National Institute of Mental Health, the National Heart Lung and Blood Institute, and other institutes of the US National Institutes of Health, we have been able to develop measures of health literacy specifically useful with patients with HIV infection (Ownby et al., 2013) as well as more broadly with those with diverse educational and health status backgrounds.

The process of developing items for FLIGHT/VIDAS began in earnest in 2008 when our group of collaborators first met and began to develop a set of items that would have a broad focus on the categories of health literacy advanced in the 2004 Institute of Medicine (IOM) report, *Health Literacy: A Prescription to End Confusion* (Nielsen-Bohlman et al., 2004), while evaluating the dimensions of literacy developed in previous assessments by the Educational Test Service and the National Adult Literacy Survey (Kirsch, 2001; Kirsch, Jungeblut, Jenkins, & Kolstad, 2002). Our group created items designed to assess participants' knowledge in the categories proposed in the IOM report (see the left column in Table 3-1 on page 30) in the prose, document, and quantitative formats (column headings). Examples of item targets are presented in the table. Once written, items were translated into the software program chosen to present items to study participants and record their answers.

In addition to creating items in English, a number items were developed in Spanish and then translated into English. Items were then translated into the other language with the study team evaluating each other's translation and most often adaptation of the item content and format for its appropriateness in each language/cultural group (Acevedo et al., 2009). The initial set of 225 items was first administered to a group of English-speaking participants that allowed us to evaluate each item's quality and difficulty. Participants in this phase were systematically interviewed at the end of their participation to elicit their reactions to questions and were asked for their feedback about confusing language and the appropriateness of response options. Results from this initial pilot were then used to revise items for use in phase I.

Development

This section provides an overview of study procedures (see Figure 3-1). Test items were developed to sample a broad range of health-related content in Spanish and English. The sample on which the measure was validated was purposefully drawn from a range of abilities and backgrounds as evidenced by participants' occupations and educations. In order to accurately characterize Spanish-speaking participants, we developed a procedure to assess language dominance in Spanish-English bilinguals. Items in both languages were created to minimize the impact of regional usage and data analyses employ a combination of classical test theory (DeVellis, 2006; Gulliksen, 1950; Lord & Novick, 1968) and item response theory (Embretson & Reise, 2000) techniques.

In Phase 1, a pool of candidate items was administered to Spanish and English speakers, with approximately one-half of each group aged 50 years or older. Items were screened for difficulty and discrimination (correlation with total score) and for age- and language-associated differential item functioning, or DIF (see section on differential functioning later in this chapter for a more detailed explanation). The original pool of items was then reduced and some new items were written to enhance the total scale's range of content and difficulty. In Phase 2, items developed

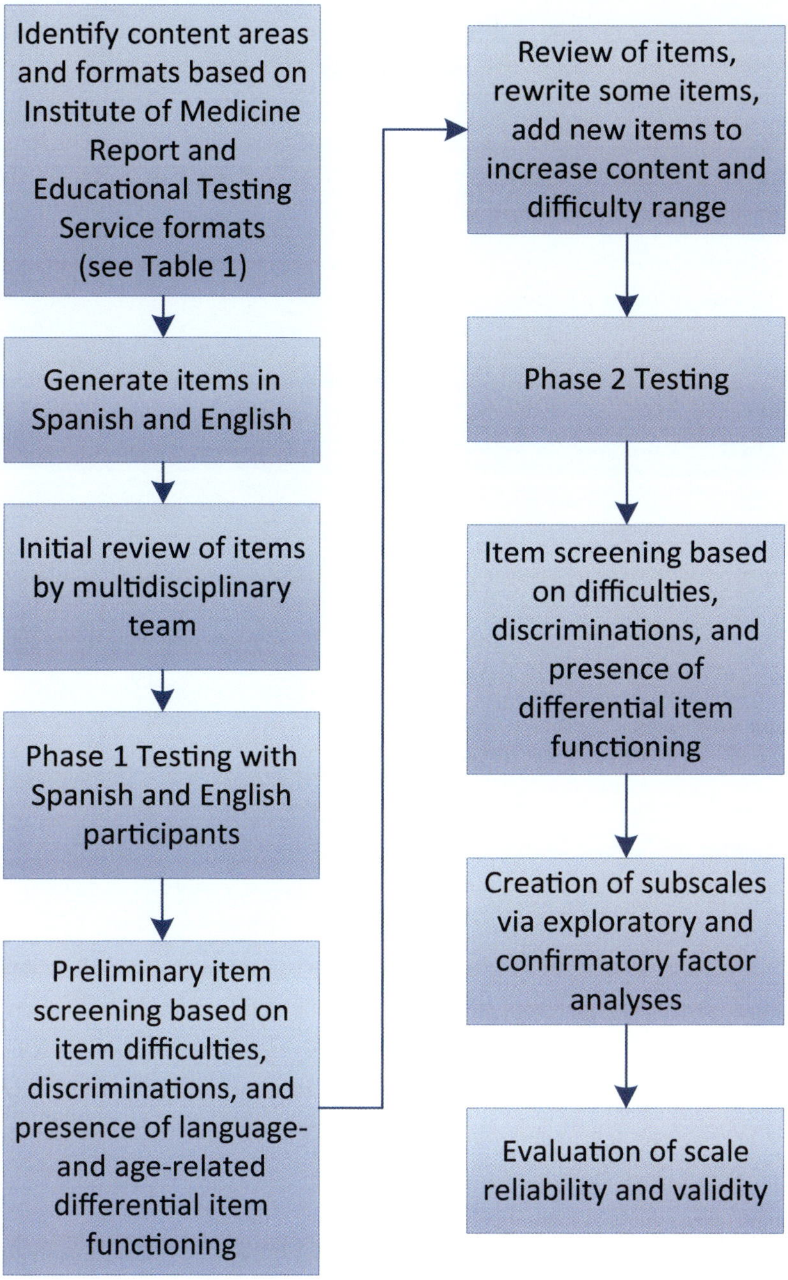

Figure 3-1. FLIGHT/VIDAS Development Process

Table 3-1. Item content examples by IOM report domains and ETS formats (from Ownby et al, 2013; reprinted with permission)

Goals of Health Literacy	Prose
Health promotion	Read a passage on exercise and identify desirable duration of exercise
Understand health information	Read a passage on risk factors for diabetes and identify relevant behaviors that would reduce someone's risk
Apply health information	After being provided with information on physical activity guidelines, identify appropriate exercise duration and frequencies
Navigate the health care system	After reading an informational brochure, be able to describe how specific health care services are covered by an insurance program
Participate in encounters with health care professionals	After viewing a video of a person's encounter with a physician providing a new medicine, identify information provided by the physician about dosage and schedule
Give informed consent	After reading information about a colonoscopy, describe the risks and benefits of the procedure

Document	Quantitative
Make menu choices based on fat and sodium guidelines	Calculate the number of grams of fat in a package of a product given a per serving value
Given a checklist of risk factors for diabetes, be able to complete a checklist of risk factors for the disease	Given information on normal and abnormal blood glucose levels, identify normal and abnormal levels
Given narrative information on exercise frequency and intensity, complete an exercise log.	Calculate the number of calories used during exercise give a table of exercises, times, and values;
Review information from a table on dates and times for applying for specific health care benefits	Calculate relative costs of two insurance plans
After viewing a video describing how to apply for long term care insurance, fill out an application	After viewing a video that presents information on desirable weights, calculate one's own body mass index
After viewing a video that presents information on informed consent for a clinical study, describe its risks and benefits.	Given a graphical representation of the probability of a medication side effect, correctly identify how likely its occurrence will be.

in Phase 1 were administered to an age-stratified sample of community-dwelling English and Spanish speakers along with measures chosen to help establish the new scale's validity, including other measures of health literacy, health-related quality of life, health status, and health service utilization.

Computer Delivered Format

In order to ensure that the resulting measure would be inexpensive and easily deployed, it was developed using off-the-shelf touchscreen computers that were readily available and reasonably priced (HP TouchSmart®; Hewlett-Packard Corporation, Palo Alto, CA). These computers had touch screens running the Windows® operating system (20 inch diagonal measurement) and include self-contained speakers that allowed participants to hear all items as they were presented. In another project, we had done extensive user testing with the general format of touch screen interface, iteratively testing the interface, modifying it in response to user comments, and then retesting it (Ownby, Waldrop-Valverde, Caballero, & Jacobs, 2012). In Phase 1, we used the previously developed touchscreen format. Interviews after each participant completed the phase 1 focused on possible usability and navigation issues as well as on the format and content of the questions. Any issues that arose were addressed before using the item in Phase 2.

Item Development

A framework for item development was created based on the domains of literacy skills needed for health as outlined in the 2004 Institute of Medicine report (Nielsen-Bohlman, Panzer, & Kindig, 2004). For each of the seven health-related goals listed in the Report (left column in Table 3–1, pages 30-31) items were created in one of the three formats commonly used in assessing literacy–prose, document, and quantitative (Kirsch et al., 2002). A 7 X 3 item content matrix was created and used as a guide in item development (Table 3-1). Candidate items were developed by individual team members and reviewed by the entire team. Development team members represented a wide range of health professions including medicine, nursing, social work, pharmacy, and psychology. Each team member had extensive experience in clinical work and thus was familiar with the types of clinical problems encountered by patients in obtaining health care. The lead investigator (RO) also had extensive experience with psychometric scale development. The team included a psychologist with a strong background in multicultural and multilingual assessment (AA) who also had published multiple articles on psychometric assessment. Other members of the team were also experienced in patient education and assessment.

Some items were first created in Spanish and then translated into English, while others were created in English and translated. A guiding principle in item development was to create items that would be culturally and linguistically equivalent rather than creating word-for-word translations (Acevedo et al., 2009). From the project's inception, word and item selection were focused on use of high-frequency words and terms to ensure that participants would understand all questions. Care was taken to use words in both languages that would be understood by persons of varying socioeconomic and educational levels and that were not specific to regions or nations.

Items developed within the 7 x 3 content matrix (Table 3-1) targeted the component skills of literacy (conceptual knowledge, listening and speaking, writing, reading, and numeracy) as outlined in the IOM report. For example, to assess conceptual knowledge, items that tapped basic health facts were created (e.g., "Hemoglobin A1C measures which of the following?"). Listening comprehension was assessed using 60-90 second videos of simulated interactions with health care providers or presentations of health information. For example, one video showed an encounter in which a patient was given a new medication and directions for its use, and another simulated a TV news presentation on finding health information on the Internet. After viewing, participants responded to multiple choice questions. It was not possible to directly assess participants' oral expression skills, but questions were created that presented problems that could only be solved by communicating with providers (e.g., "Arthur doesn't understand what the doctor says. What can he do?").

Written expression was assessed as document literacy through questions evaluating participants' ability to complete materials such as insurance forms. Navigating the health care system included interpreting hospital maps; some documents and maps included items that asked participants to respond by tapping on the appropriate area of the screen (e.g., "Tap on the area where you would find information on how to use toothpaste with a 4 year old"). Reading comprehension was assessed through questions about passages of varying difficulty levels, and numeracy was assessed through items demanding reading, arithmetic computation and decision making based on probabilities. Approximately 10-12 items were created for each element in the item content matrix resulting in 225 candidate items.

Phase 1: Initial Item Testing

This base group of items was administered to 73 English– and 69 Spanish–speaking participants. Language dominance of Spanish-speaking participants who indicated that they also spoke English was assessed by comparing their performance on the relative proficiency indices (RPI) of the reading and listening comprehension subtests of the Woodcock-Johnson (English) and the Woodcock-Muñoz (Spanish) Psycho-Educational Batteries (Woodcock, McGrew, & Mather, 2007; Woodcock, Muñoz-Sandoval, McGrew, & Mather, 2007). Level of acculturation was assessed using the Marin Acculturation Scale (Marin, Sabogal, Marin, Otero-Sabogal, & Perez-Stable, 1987). Most participants showed clear superiority in one language or the other (i.e., more than one standard deviation difference in RPI scores), including those who indicated they had proficiency in both languages. Only those participants who showed clear evidence of greater proficiency in Spanish completed the Spanish assessments. The importance of actually assessing Hispanic participants' language skills is underscored by a study that showed that Hispanics who state they are fluent in English may function at lower levels compared to native English speakers

(Aguirre et al., 2005).

Almost half of each language group was 50 years of age or older (29 of 73 English and 30 of 69 Spanish speakers) allowing for the assessment of language- and age-related DIF. As discussed above, we believed that this issue was important in light of our finding that almost one-half of the items on the reading comprehension scale of the TOFHLA showed evidence of age-related differential item functioning, or DIF. After responding to all items, participants completed interviews during which items were reviewed with them for problems in clarity and to assess whether the items actually measured what was intended. Initial analyses were completed using jMetrik (Meyer, 2014), assessing item difficulties, discriminations (item-total correlations), and the presence of DIF. The Mantel-Haenszel chi-square statistic as well as the Educational Testing Service grading system were used to evaluate DIF, supplemented by review of nonparametric item response curves.

In creating the final item pool for further study, some items were eliminated due language-related DIF, while other items were rewritten after team consultation. No items showed substantial age-related DIF, supporting our decision to avoid using the cloze response procedure used in other measures, as it may bias items against older individuals (Ownby & Waldrop-Valverde, 2013; Ownby, Acevedo, Waldrop-Valverde, & Jacobs, 2014). A number of items were either low or mid-range in difficulty; many of these were eliminated when their content or format duplicated other items. Data from interviews were used to rewrite items when participants indicated that an item was confusing or when the interviews showed that the item did not actually assess its target skill. Several new items were created in this phase in order to broaden the range of content covered and provide items with greater difficulties. Although these items were not subjected to the same developmental testing as with other items in Phase 1, they were be assessed for psychometric characteristics prior to inclusion in the group of items tested in Phase 2.

Phase 2: Further Development

The purpose of phase 2 was to evaluate item characteristics and validate the measure by assessing its relations to other measures of health literacy and participants' health. A purposive sample with a range of abilities (based on education and occupation) was recruited over specific age groups by decades from the 20 to 70s and older (see Tables 3–3. 3–4, & 3–5). We judged that this strategy was most likely to be the most efficient approach to obtain optimal item statistics with a relatively small sample (Orlando, 2004; Wingersky & Lord, 1984). Interested participants were first screened for cognitive status using the Short Portable Mental Status Questionnaire and paragraphs from the Wechsler Memory Scale using cut off scores previously developed in a study of computer use in elderly participants. Participants were screened for intact vision and auditory abilities using a visual screener and auditory comprehension of material presented over headphones calibrated using a handheld decibel meter (Extech Model 407730, Extech Instruments, Waltham MA). Spanish-speaking participants were recruited from several different national backgrounds including the countries of Central and South America and the Caribbean, as well as the US and Mexico. The language of assessment was determined as described previously, using the procedure developed in Phase 1. Participants first completed the language preference subscale of the Marin Acculturation Scale. When participants indicated significant use of both languages and language dominance was not clear, the determination was supplemented with additional testing to determine language used.

In addition to the new health literacy items, participants completed a battery of established health literacy measures (TOFHLA in both Spanish and English; REALM or SAHLSA, the self-report questions developed by Chew et al. (2004), and literacy- and numeracy-related academic skills and basic cognitive abilities. They also provided information on their health status, health-related quality of life, and health service utilization. Participants completed assessments in two sessions (individually-administered cognitive and health literacy measures in one, questionnaires and the health literacy measures administered by touch screen computer in the other) with order of administration of each session randomly counterbalanced to account for order effects. Because of the length of assessment sessions, participants completed both sessions either in a single day (during which they took at least a one-hour break for lunch) or on two days. Measures were selected to allow the evaluation of the relation of the new measure to existing assessments of health literacy, basic cognitive skills, relevant academic skills such as reading and math skills, and health status variables.

Who Were Our Participants?

Since we wanted to develop a measure of health literacy that would be useful in both Spanish and English speakers, we wanted to better understand how well our bilingual participants spoke English and Spanish. We focused on ensuring that persons assessed in Spanish were actually competent in Spanish through a screening and testing procedure that, when their language backgrounds were not clear, evaluated with objective tests the language proficiency of individuals who indicated that they were proficient in both English and Spanish.

The screening procedure for all participants included a question about whether they spoke any other languages in addition to English. Persons who indicated that they spoke more than one language were asked about their language use at home and with friends using questions from the Marin et al. (1987) cultural assessment tool. While the majority of potential participants indicated that they primarily used English or Spanish in their daily lives, some reported a balance. Those whose responses suggested significant competence in both languages were tested using a procedure developed during Phase 1 of the project. Individuals whose linguistic status was unclear were therefore asked to complete both timed listening and reading assessments in each language. The majority of participants, even those who indicated that they felt they could complete F/V in English, clearly fell in a specific language group based on their responses. It is important to note that many individuals who initially indicated that

Table 3-2. Participant Gender, Language and Age

		Age Group						
		18-29	30-39	40-49	50-59	60-69	70+	Total
English	Men	15	13	14	24	14	14	94
	Women	18	22	20	18	26	45	149
	Total	33	35	34	42	40	59	243
Spanish	Men	14	11	21	13	11	24	94
	Women	12	19	34	36	23	32	156
	Total	26	30	55	49	34	56	250
Total	Men	29	24	35	37	W25	38	188
	Women	30	41	54	54	49	77	305
	Total	59	65	89	91	74	115	493

Table 3-3. Participant Race, Language and Age

		Age in Decades						
		18-29	30-39	40-49	50-59	60-69	70+	Total
English	White	15	9	10	22	22	44	122
	Black	18	26	24	20	18	15	121
	Total	33	35	34	42	40	59	243
Spanish	White	26	30	55	49	34	56	250
	Total	26	30	55	49	34	56	250
Total	White	41	39	65	71	56	100	372
	Black	18	26	24	20	18	15	121
	Total	59	65	89	91	74	115	493

Table 3-4. Means and Standard Deviations for Age, Education, and Health Literacy Measures by Language and Age

			Age	Education	TOFHLA Num	TOFHLA Read	REALM	SAHLSA
English	18-29 N=25	Mean	23.33	12.82	48.00	47.21	63.18	
		SD	3.92	2.13	2.29	2.04	3.72	
	30-39 N=35	Mean	33.71	13.47	47.74	46.37	61.26	
		SD	2.78	2.20	3.54	3.71	9.24	
	40-49 N=35	Mean	45.00	12.22	46.12	45.00	59.41	
		SD	2.76	2.25	4.01	5.06	11.90	
	50-59 N=42	Mean	54.02	12.90	47.14	44.93	61.24	
		SD	2.97	2.32	3.52	5.93	8.09	
	60-69 N=40	Mean	63.93	13.34	47.32	44.49	61.68	
		SD	2.89	2.82	4.65	8.18	9.26	
	70+ N=59	Mean	77.15	13.79	47.19	45.42	63.12	
		SD	4.79	2.47	4.42	6.16	8.78	
	Total N=243	Mean	52.91	13.16	47.24	45.51	61.78	
		SD	18.91	2.43	3.90	5.70	8.84	
Spanish	18-29 N=26	Mean	24.08	11.92	44.42	46.65		44.38
		SD	3.61	3.17	7.27	2.77		4.63
	30-39 N=30	Mean	34.97	12.07	43.70	45.03		45.17
		SD	2.57	3.48	6.20	7.29		4.85
	40-49 N=55	Mean	44.73	12.65	43.40	44.94		45.91
		SD	2.98	2.38	6.51	5.20		4.82
	50-59 N=49	Mean	54.02	12.02	42.73	42.65		44.96
		SD	2.68	3.29	6.56	9.04		5.50
	60-69 N=34	Mean	64.29	11.18	41.32	39.21		45.74
		SD	2.73	2.97	7.23	10.10		3.45
	70+ N=56	Mean	78.38	9.68	39.70	31.88		43.22
		SD	6.06	3.93	7.15	12.47		5.89
	Total N=250	Mean	53.43	11.52	42.30	40.96		44.86
		SD	17.84	3.39	6.94	10.25		5.09

they could complete the measure in English clearly had better Spanish language skills. Characteristics of the participants are presented in Tables 3–3, 3–4, and 3–5.

Assessing Validity

Several strategies were used to assess the validity of the new measure. Construct validity was assessed through a series of exploratory and confirmatory factor analyses that assessed the dimensions of health literacy assessed by the items. The factor structure of the measure was assessed separately for English and Spanish speakers via exploratory and confirmatory approaches, and the equivalence of the measure's factor structure in both language groups was evaluated.

Classical test theory item analyses were used to assess item difficulties and their relation to the measure's underlying core dimension. From the initial item pool evaluated in phase 1, a subset of items were chosen for further evaluation in Phase 2 based on a range of item content and difficulty as well as the absence of differential item functioning. Final item

Table 3-5. Tests of improvement of model fit for exploratory factor models with 1 to 6 factors

Comparison			χ^2	df	*p*
1-factor	against	2-factor	521.224	97	0.0000
2-factor	against	3-factor	330.075	96	0.0000
3-factor	against	4-factor	227.275	95	0.0000
4-factor	against	5-factor	144.246	94	0.0007
5-factor	against	6-factor	135.577	93	0.0026

Table 3-6. Fit statistics for exploratory factor models with 1 to 6 factors

	χ^2	df	*p*	RMSEA	CFI	TLI
1	5627.32	4655	0.000	0.021	0.936	0.935
2	5077.05	4558	0.000	0.015	0.966	0.964
3	4713.66	4462	0.004	0.011	0.983w	0.982
4	4502.78	4367	0.074	0.008	0.991	0.990
5	4372.94	4273	0.140	0.007	0.993	0.993
6	4247.94	4180	0.228	0.006	0.996	0.995

analyses after data collection was complete allowed the verification of scales provisionally developed based on phase 1 data and interim analyses of phase 2 data.

DIF between English and Spanish speakers was assessed at the initial stage of item development, after pilot testing the items, and at the end of data collection. As the first two stages of measure development, items were found that functioned differentially in English and Spanish speakers. At the final analysis, only one item remained with significant DIF; it was eliminated. Scale equivalence in English and Spanish was evaluated using item response theory linking and equating procedures available in jMetrik software (Meyer, 2014).

Exploratory Factor Analyses

Factor analysis is a way to identify dimensions that underlie responses to a group of test questions. For example, a group of people could be asked questions that assess their skills with words and at the same time ask them to answer questions that assess their ability to visualize geometric forms in their head. If their responses were factor analyzed, we

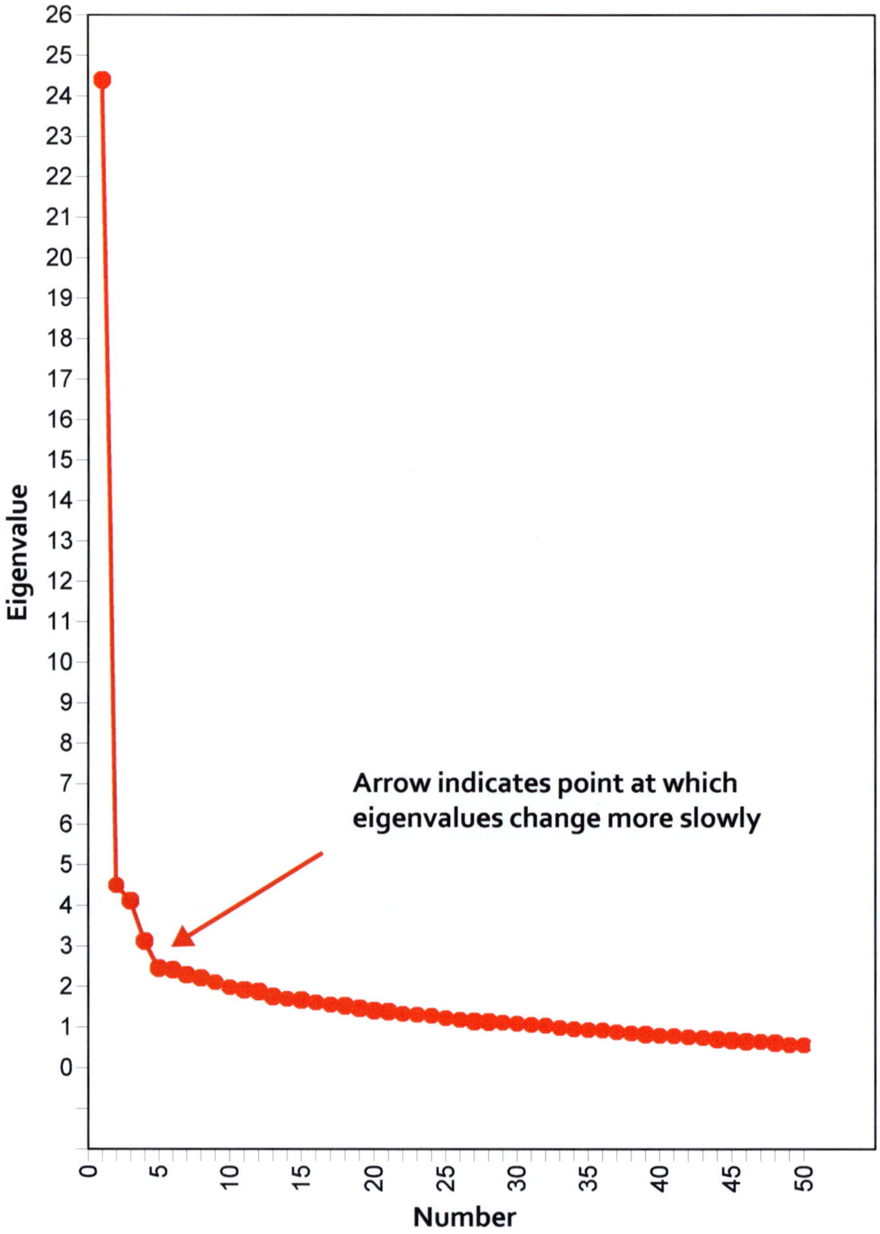

Figure 3-2. Scree plot of eigenvalues for the combined sample of English and Spanish speakers

would probably find that the word-related items were closely related to each other (i.e., highly correlated), and the items about geometric forms would be closely related to each other as well. The two sets of items would be related to each other as well, but not as closely. Factor analysis would allow a determination of how closely each of the questions is related to underlying verbal or visuospatial abilities. The analysis results in a estimate called a factor loading of how closely each item is releated to the underlying ability dimensions.

The 98 items administered to participants in Phase 2 were subjected to exploratory factor analyses using routines available for analysis of categorical variables available in MPlus (Muthén & Muthén, 2012). The number of factors in the items was determined by inspection of the scree plot of eigenvalues (Figure 3-2), statistical tests of the improvement of factor model fit with larger number of factors (Table 3-5), and assessment of how well factor models with different numbers of dimensions meaningfully fit the data. The scree plot (Figure 3-2) shows that the size of eigenvalues extracted became smaller and tended to change in very small amounts after four factors were extracted (arrow in Figure3-2).

Statistical tests of the improvement in model fit with increasing numbers of factors are presented in Table 3-5. Model fit improved with each additional factor up to six. Fit statistics for the exploratory factor analytic models are presented in Table 3-6. A four-factor model resulted in a non-significant χ^2 value, indicating that the model with this number of factors fit the data well. Other values listed in the table are the RMSEA (root mean square error of approximation), CFI (comparative fit index), and TLI (Tucker-Lewis index). Values of the RMSEA less than 0.05 are generally considered to indicate good model fit, while values of the CFI and TLI greater than 0.95 are considered desirable. It can be seen that the four-factor model met these criteria. Finally, even though five- and six-factor models showed improved fit (Table 3-5), evaluation of the content of these two models showed that only a small number of items were included in these factors and that they did not represent important dimensions of FLIGHT/VIDAS.

Table 3-7. Fit statistics for four-factor confirmatory models by language group and equivalence models

Model	χ^2	df	*p*	RMSEA	CFI	TLI
English	2892.03	2685	0.0028	0.018	0.964	0.963
Spanish	2855.76	2685	0.0110	0.016	0.972	0.971
Combined	3159.03	2685	< 0.001	0.019	0.970	0.969
Configural	5749.42	5370	0.0002	0.017	0.968	0.968
Scalar	5897.31	5442	< 0.001	0.018	0.962	0.961

Exploratory analyses were also completed in the English and Spanish samples separately. Results of exploratory factor models were similar in both language group on examination of fit and factor loadings. This interpretation was subsequently tested in confirmatory analyses.

Confirmatory Factor Analyses

These exploratory analyses allowed to us to develop a model of the factors underlying the FV variables for further testing in confirmatory factor analysis (CFA) models. EFA results suggested the appropriateness of a four-factor model based on inspection of the plot of the eigenvalues and change in chi-square values for models with progressively larger number of factors. A four-factor model appeared to fit our data well based on RMSEA, CFI, and TLI values.

These four factors represented (1) ***general health literacy*** (reading passages and understanding documents), (2) ***numeracy*** (arithmetic calculations and understanding probability and risk, (3) ***conceptual health knowledge,*** and (4) ***listening***. A four factor model based on these dimensions was therefore created and tested. Tests of this model (Table 3-7) showed that it fit the data of separate language-group samples as well as the combined sample of English and Spanish speakers well, although model lack of fit was still present as indicated by significant χ^2 values. Indexes that show the four-factor model fit the combined data well included the RMSEA, all of which are less than 0.05 indicating adequate fit, and the CFI and TLI values all of which are greater than 0.95 indicating adequate fit.

English and Spanish Scales

A key goal of the F/V project was to create a measure that would be useful and equivalent in both English and Spanish. Throughout the project this goal was kept in mind, from the initial conception of the project through item development and finally in data analyses. The equivalence of the F/V scales were assessed in three ways: (1) assessment of the equivalence of the measure's factor structure in English and Spanish; (2) evaluation of all items for indications of differential item functioning; and (3) testing the relation of the HL scale in both languages through item response theory scale linking. These complementary approaches provided an overall assessment of the extent to which the scale can be used with persons who speak either language and the perhaps most importantly compare scores between groups.

Factor Structure Equivalence

An important question is the extent to which the dimensions of health literacy represented in FLIGHT/VIDAS are the same in English and Spanish speakers. This question was assessed in confirmatory analyses that evaluated, first, the extent to which the factor structure was the same (even if the language groups were different on level of performance or in the ways that each item measures the dimensions it's related to) and then a stricter comparison that these same issues were the same in the two groups. Fit statistics for the four-factor models for the English- and Spanish-speaking and for the configural and scalar models are presented in Table 3-7. It can be seen that all models were associated with significant χ^2 values, suggesting that they did not fit the data exactly. All models, however, were associated with RMSEA values less than 0.05 (suggesting adequate fit)

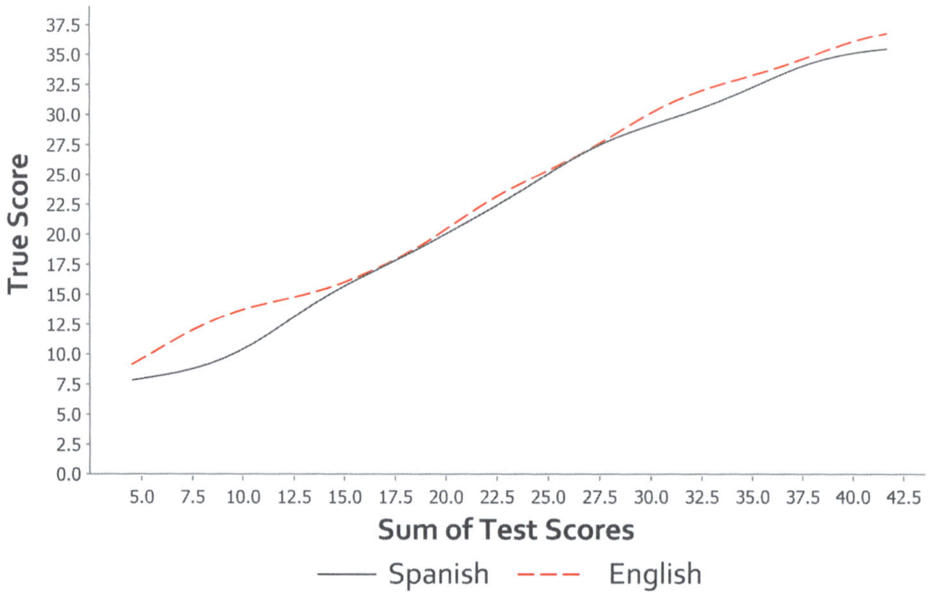

Figure 3-3. Test characteristic curves

and with CFI and TLI values greater than 0.95 (again suggesting adequate model fit). The fit of the scalar invariance model was significantly poorer than that of the configural invariance model (difference in χ^2 [df = 72] = 154.80, $p < 0.001$), although it can be noted that the fit of both invariance models was adequate as evaluated by the three fit indexes.

Differential Item Functioning

Differential item functioning (DIF) exists when a test item is more or less difficult for members of one group compared to another even though they have the same overall ability. Testing for DIF is important, since its presence implies that one group's scores on a measure may be different from another's because of the measurement tool itself rather than because of real differences in what the measure is believed to assess. Because of our concern for developing a measure that would be widely useful, we tested for DIF related to language and age because we had found evidence of age-related DIF in the TOFHLA (Ownby & Waldrop-Valverde, 2013; Ownby et al., 2014). DIF related to language group was assessed at the initial stage of item development, after pilot testing the items, and at the end of data collection. DIF analyses are usually based in item response theory (IRT) analyses and require large sample sizes. For this development project we used a nonparametric approach to DIF analysis available in the jMetrk software (Meyer, 2014). This strategy allows an assessment of between-group DIF by plotting item characteristics for each group. When DIF exists in an item, there is a discrepancy between the difficulty of an item in each group for individuals of the same overall ability. In F/V development, we assessed language, age, and education related DIF in phase 1 and in selecting items for phase 2. The final scale eliminated all items with substantial DIF. The test characteristic curve for the final 40-item scale is presented in Figure 3-3. It can be seen that the overall curve for the two groups is essentially equivalent, although the scale may be slightly more difficult for lower ability Spanish speakers.

Scale Equivalence and Linking

Two scale are equivalent if they measure the same thing; in the case of the FLIGHT/VIDAS project, we were primarily interested in evaluating how performance on the scales of FLIGHT/VIDAS was the same among English and Spanish speakers. This assessment was important because it would allow users to assess differences in health literacy between groups of English and Spanish speakers, and to date, no measure of health literacy had been shown equivalent in the two language groups. (Even though the TOFHLA has both English and Spanish versions, as of this date no readily-identifiable study has demonstrated its equivalence in the two language groups. In fact, the reading items of the Spanish version are not the same as in the English version, making the two measure's equivalence unlikely).

Table 3-8. Computer Administered FLIGHT/VIDAS scales

Scale	Example
General Health Literacy (HL): The ability to read and complete mental operations on health care information, including identify relevant information in prose, documents, and figures (39 items).	***Prose:*** After reading instructions for laboratory test preparation, correctly identify appointment time. ***Document:*** Correctly identify fields in an insurance form; Use an electronic device on a Web page to calculate body mass index.
Numeracy (NUM): The application of quantitative skills including arithmetic operations and appraisal of relations among numeric concepts such as ratios and percentages (24 items).	Correctly identify meaning of terms related to probability; Correctly identify number of grams of fat consumed in a meal based on values in a table.
Conceptual Knowledge (Experimental Scale; FACT): Demonstrate understanding of specific concepts related to health care (14 items).	Correctly identify the organ treated by a medical specialist such as a cardiologist
Listening Comprehension (Experimental Scale; LIS): The ability to acquire and remember information presented orally (13 items).	After viewing a video of a clinician giving information about participation in a clinical research study, correctly identify treatment alternatives.

This table originally appeared in Ownby et al. (2013). Reprinted with permission of the publisher.

Scale equivalence in English and Spanish speakers was evaluated using IRT linking and equating procedures (Meyer, 2014). In this approach, IRT analyses assessed item difficulties in the two groups and then compared them so that scores on the scales in one language group could predict scores in the other. Various models compare group performances, predicting the mean or combining the mean with the scale variance. All models suggested that the HL scales in English and Spanish were equivalent. Equations to predict scores on one measure based on the other each had intercepts of 1.00, consistent with minimal overall difference in level of performance between groups. Depending on the linking method, the coefficient in the regression equation relating one score to another was either zero (mean predicting mean) or very small (-0.02 for the Haebara method and -0.04 for the Stocking-Lord method). While this explanation may seem technical, the conclusion to be drawn from these analyses is straightforward. Scores on the English HL scale are very similar to those on the Spanish version of the scale.

Scales

The factor analytic work combined with classical test theory analyses of item characteristics provided the information needed to choose items that would allow us to reduce the 98 items tested to a smaller number that could be assembled into scales measuring specific dimensions of health literacy. The dimensions of health literacy were described above, and the final computer-administered scales are described in Table 3-8. We also received requests from a number of potential users to create a measure that could be hand administered and scored, and our discussions with a number of persons at various conferences where we presented data on F/V development led us to believe that a short measure that could be used for screening would also be useful to a number of clinicians and researchers. We therefore created two additional subscales of F/V using items that did not require computer administration.

Computer Administered Scales (Table 3-8)

As exploratory factor analyses suggested that the FLIGHT/VIDAS items included a dimension of general health literacy reflecting an individual's ability to extract meaning from written texts and documents. This scale was named General Health Literacy and referred to as HL. Another scale reflected the ability to use quantitative concepts in health care decision making or tracking of health status and is interpreted as reflecting numeracy (NUM). Consistent with our plan to develop a number of items that assessed conceptual knowledge of health, a subgroup of items was judged to reflect conceptual knowledge as contrasted with the ability to use more complex mental operations; this scale is referred to as FACT. Finally, a number of items assessed the ability to acquire information presented in video simulations of health care encounters, health-related TV news story, information related to providing informed consent, and instructions on healthy diet. This is the Listening Comprehension scale, or LIS.

Pencil and Paper Scales

As discussed earlier in Chapter 1, although our primary intention was to develop a scale that was computer administered and scored, ongoing feedback from potential users has indicated a strong interest in being able to administered F/V individually without a computer or Internet access. Given the number of questions and the diverse formats of items tested in Phase 2, it was possible create a paper and pencil version of the measure that could be hand scored. In creating this version of the scale, we created test materials that were replicas of the computer screens used in the computer-administered version of the scale. Please see the F/V web site for information about obtaining test materials (www.flightvidas.org).

A question may arise with respect of the validity of this administration strategy since it varies from the approach jused in scale development and validation. We note that Chesser et al. (2014) compared computer-administered and individually-administered versions of the S-TOFHLA. Results of this study showed that the computer version was essentially identical to that individually-administered version. Results of this study were con-

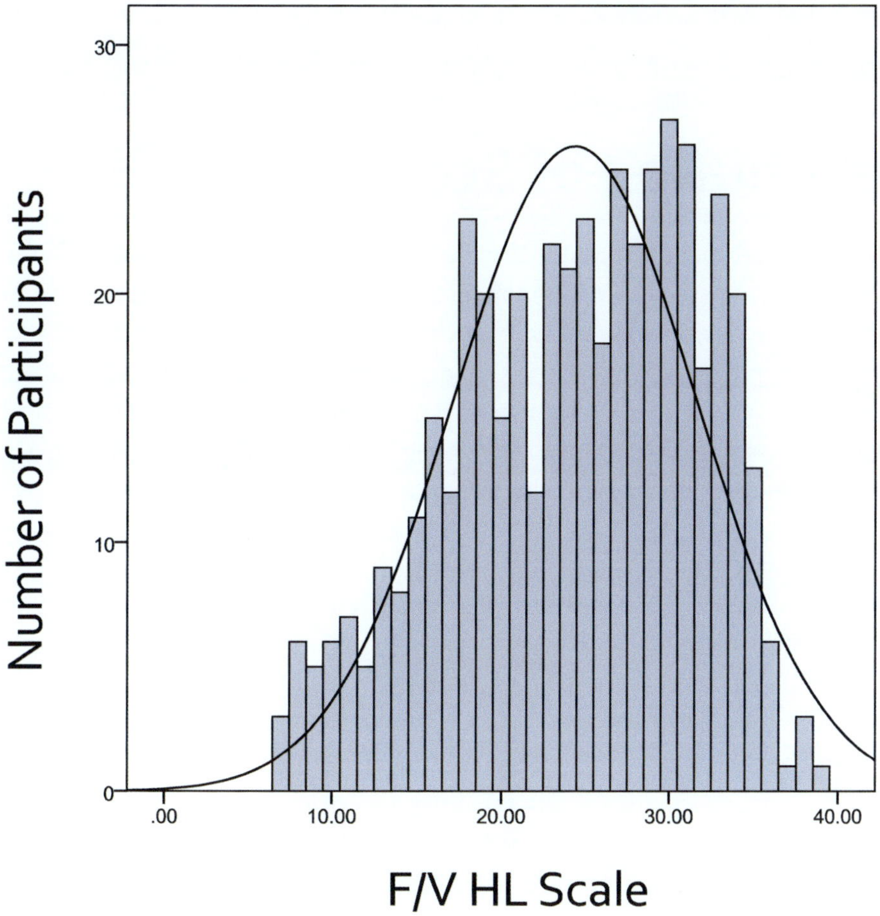

Figure 3-4. Distribution of scores on the 40-item F/V General Health Literacy scale

sistent with results of multiple other studies of computer-administered versions of paper and pencil scales. These have shown that computer-administered versions of measures are, in general, functionally equivalent as long as test materials and order of administration are the same (Gwaltney, Shields, & Shiffman, 2008; Millsap, 2000). The 20 items of the HL paper scale were selected to reflect a moderate range of difficulties, a range of content, and to consistently have high item discriminations. This strategy would make the scale maximally useful across settings (e.g., healthcare, general health promotion) and include not only reading but also document and numeracy tasks. Information on these scales' reliability and validity in presented in Chapter 4.

Distribution of Scores

An important problem with the use of the TOFHLA, S-TOFHLA, REALM, and SAHLSA in research on health literacy with normal groups is the finding that a very large number of persons will attain perfect or near perfect scores on these measures–this is often termed "ceiling effect." In a study using the S-TOFHLA in metropolitan Detroit with a substantial number of lower-income participants, for example, 96.7% of 599 participants had a score that was classified as "adequate" health literacy (Schwartz et al., 2013).

Similarly, in the F/V final sample, slightly more than 25% of the sample achieved scores of 96 or greater (of a possible total TOFHLA score of 100), and even though nearly 50% of the sample scored below the 8th grade level on an individually-administered and nationally-normed standardized reading measure (the Woodcock-Johnson or Woodcock-Muñoz Passage Comprehension subtest), only 5% of our participants scored at the inadequate level of the full-length TOFHLA while another 7.6% of our participants scored in the marginal range.

In statistical terms, the skewness statistic for the TOFHLA total score was -1.88, indicating that the distribution of scores was highly skewed. In fact, nearly 60% of our participants had scores of 90 or greater. By contrast, the distribution of scores for the F/V scale was approximately symmetric, with a skewness statistic of -0.38 indicating a small departure from normality. The distribution of F/V General Health Literacy scale scores is presented in Figure 3-4. The F/V scale clearly has a much larger range of scores, allowing a more precise assessment of health literacy across a broad range of abilities.

4 Reliability and Validity

Overview

Multiple strategies are available to evaluate the reliability and validity of a measure like F/V. In evaluating the F/V scales, we assessed their internal reliability using a standard index, Cronbach's α (alpha). We evaluated validity in several ways, as the scales' correlations with other measures and its ability to discriminate among groups of people who reported difficulties in understanding written health information.

Reliability

A standard strategy to evaluate the reliability of a measure is to calculate an index of the scale's internal consistency. Probably the most common measure of this sort is Cronbach's α. Acceptable values for this measure vary depending on the purpose for which a scale is used, but most authors suggest that a value of 0.80 and greater can be considered acceptable. Table 4-1 present the α values for each of the FLIGHT/VIDAS scales for language groups and for the combined sample. The standard scales for the measure, HL, NUM, and Paper each have acceptable levels of internal reliability as assessed by Cronbach's α. The FACT and LIS scales have borderline unacceptable reliabilities and should be considered useful in research pending further development.

Table 4-1. Cronbach's α for subscales

	HL40[a]	Paper	NUM	FACT[b]	LIS[b]
English	0.87	0.88	0.88	0.73	0.64
Spanish	0.85	0.89	0.86	0.61	0.56
Combined	0.87	0.89	0.88	0.69	0.58

[a]HL40 = 40-item general health literacy scale; Paper = 20-item paper and pencil scale; NUM = health numeracy scale; FACT = conceptual knowledge scale; LIS = listening scale.
[b]Because of low reliability values, the FACT and LIS scales should be considered experimental.

Validity

Face validity

As more extensively discussed in Chapter 3, the items used in creating FLIGHT/VIDAS were developed from a matrix of contents and formats developed by a panel of experts who created a definition of the goals of health literacy. The interested reader can consult Table 3-1 to further assess the extent to which F/V scales have adequate face validity.

Convergent validity

In this strategy, validity is assessed as a scale's relation to other measures of the same construct. In F/V, the full version of the Test of Functional Health Literacy in Adults (TOFHLA) was administered in either English or Spanish to all participants. English-speaking participants also completed the Rapid Estimate of Adult Literacy in Medicine (REALM) while Spanish speakers completed the Short Assessment of Health Literacy in Spanish-speaking Adults (SAHLSA). Correlations of the scales of FLIGHT/

Table 4-2. Subscale correlations with TOFHLA

	Paper	NUM	FACT	LIS	TOF R	TOF N
HL40	0.88[a]	0.79	0.76	0.68	0.65	0.49
Paper		0.90	0.54	0.66	0.68	0.53
NUM			0.53	0.57	0.58	0.49
FACT				0.43	0.44	0.36
LIS					0.55	0.37
TOF R						0.53

[a]All *ps* < 0.001; TOF R = TOFHLA Reading Scale; TOF N = TOFHLA Numeracy Scale;HL40 = 40-item general health literacy scale; HL20 = 20-item general health literacy scale; Paper = 25-item paper and pencil version; NUM = health numeracy scale; FACT = conceptual knowledge scale; LIS = listening scale.

VIDAS with these other measures are presented in Tables 4-2 and 4-3.

The convergent validity of F/V scales was also evaluated by assessing its relation to measures of health-related quality of life (MOS SF-36), self-report of health status (number and frequency of physical symptoms and number of diagnosed health conditions), an overall measure of health quality of life derived from the SF–36 scales (EQ5D) and a measure of depressive symptoms, the Center for Epidemiological Studies Depression Scale (CES-D). The values in Table 4-4 show that F/V scales were significantly related to these variables at a level similar to or greater than the TOFHLA Total score.

Known groups validity

Known groups validity refers to the ability of a measure to discriminate among groups defined by some external criterion. In the case of F/V, we

Table 4-3. Subscale correlations with REALM, SAHLSA, and academic measures

	REALM	SAHLSA	Reading	Arithmetic
HL40	0.42[a]	0.46	0.56	0.52
Paper	0.45	0.36	0.53	0.55
NUM	0.40	0.25	0.56	0.63
FACT	0.36	0.46	0.52	0.41
LIS	0.28	0.36	0.42	0.33

[a]*p* for all correlations in this table < 0.001.
Note: Only English speakers completed the REALM, while only Spanish speakers completed the SAHLSA. Reading = Woodcock-Johnson or Woodcock-Muñoz Reading Comprehension subtests; Arithmetic = Woodcock-Johnson or Woodcock-Muñoz Applied Problems subtests.

chose to evaluate this in two ways. First, groups of participants were defined by their performance on the TOFHLA, since it is one of the most widely used measures of health literacy and a number of other measures have been linked to those categories. In addition, we defined groups based on their own report of difficulties in understanding written health information using one of the questions developed by Chew et al. (2004). Results of these analyses showed statistically significant differences in F/V HL scores across groups defined by the TOFHLA categories of "Inadequate," "Marginal," and "Adequate" ($F [2, 483] = 103.51$, $p < 0.001$), and across the three self-report questions asking about difficulty in understanding written information ($F [4, 468] = 13.66$, $p < 0.001$), confidence in filling out medical forms ($F [3, 472] = 27.24$, $p < 0.001$), and reading hospital forms ($F [4, 471] = 16.02$, $p < 0.001$). Mean scores for the F/V HL scale for each level of confidence in filling out medical forms are presented in Figure 4-1.

Table 4-4. Subscale correlations with other health-related measures (TOFHLA included for comparison)

	SF Gen Health	SF Well Being	Sx	Cond	EQ5D	CESD
HL40	0.10[a]	0.21[b]	-0.18[b]	-0.15[c]	0.25[b]	-0.26[b]
Paper	0.09[d]	0.15[c]	-0.17[b]	-0.16[b]	0.24[b]	-0.22[b]
NUM	0.09[a]	0.14[a]	-0.15[c]	-0.14[a]	0.22[b]	-0.22[b]
FACT	0.09[e]	0.16[c]	-0.11[a]	-0.02[e]	0.11[a]	-0.19[b]
LIS	0.01[e]	0.13[a]	-0.09[e]	-0.12[a]	0.18[b]	-0.15[c]
TOFHLA	0.07[e]	0.12[a]	-0.15[c]	-0.18[b]	0.17[b]	0.13[a]

[a]$p < 0.05$; [b]$p < 0.001$; [c]$p = 0.001$; [d]$p = 0.05$; [e]*not significant.*
SF Gen Health = SF36 General Health; SF Well Being = SF36 Emotional Well Being ; Sx = Self-report of number and frequency of physical symptoms; Condn = number of health diagnoses; EQ5D = health quality of life index predicted from SF36; CESD = Center for Epidemiological Studies Depression Scale; TOFHLA = TOFHLA total score

Scales

The larger number of items evaluated and their diverse content and format allowed us to reduce the total number of items needed to assess health literacy while maintaining the measure's reliability and validity. Based on factor and item analyses, several briefer subscales were developed. These include the computer-administered scales derived from factor analyses as described in Chapter 3: General Health Literacy (HL), Health Numeracy (NUM), health-related conceptual knowledge (FACT), and understanding auditory health information (LIS). Because of interest

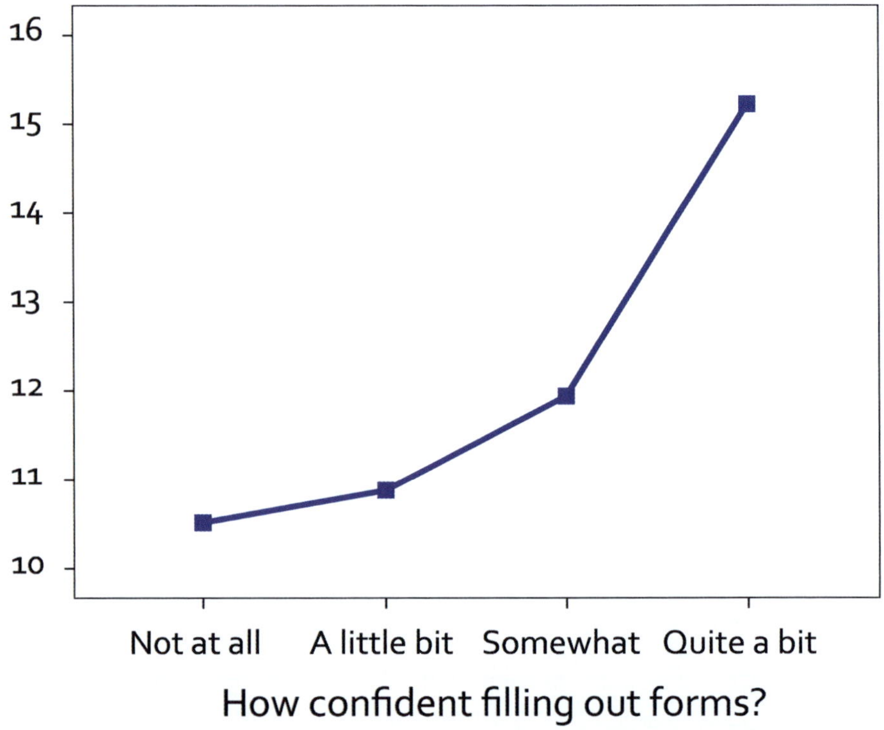

Figure 4-1. Group means for HL paper form scored across responses to question on confidence in filling out forms.

in a paper and pencil version of FLIGHT/VIDAS, a scale that included only items that could be presented in paper and pencil format (Paper) was also created. Finally, the need for a brief measure that could be used for quick screening gave rise to a ten-item screening tool, also available in paper and pencil format.

General Health Literacy (HL)

The general health literacy scale (HL) includes the best 40 items from phase 2 of the FLIGHT/VIDAS project. "Best" in this context means that they represented a broad range of content and difficulties while having a strong overall relation to the rest of the items (point biserial correlation with scale total). It includes items that evaluate reading comprehension, numeracy, conceptual knowledge, and listening.

Paper and Pencil

This scale is composed of items drawn from the HL scale that could be presented in paper and pencil format. A test booklet with these items and an answer sheet are available (go to www.flightvidas.org for information about obtaining these materials) so that this scale can be administered without a computer. In lieu of computer-delivered narration of questions, the test booklet provides directions for the individual administration of each item as the examiner reads relevant portions of each question. This procedure may be especially important for persons with low general literacy levels who may find the audio narration important in understanding questions. Because this format was not specifically validated in the original development project, norms for this scale should be interpreted cautiously, but as noted in Chapter 3, studies suggest that computer and paper and pencil measures are largely equivalent when test materials are as similar as possible in each form.

Numeracy (NUM)

This scale includes items that require mental arithmetic or understanding of probability. Many of the items ask that the person assessed read tables or figures to identify information needed to answer a question. Several questions require appraisal of probability or multi-stage arithmetic calculations to obtain a correct answer.

Conceptual Health Knowledge (FACT)

This subscale includes 14 items that only require knowledge of a specific fact about health or healthcare. None require reading extended prose or arithmetic operations. This scale has a borderline internal reliability, although it has been clearly related to important health status variables in analyses of the ASK model as discussed in Chapter 2 of this manual as well as Ownby et al. (2014). Because of its psychometric characteristics, its use should be confined to research use. It may be useful in combination with HL and NUM in understanding the extent to which a patient's functional health literacy is related to their basic academic skills in reading or mathematics or to their general knowledge about health and healthcare.

Listening Comprehension (LIS)

Items on this scale are based on questions related to the three video simulations or the audio visual slide presentation included in the original administration. This scale has a low internal reliability and is undergoing further development. In one published study (Ownby, Acevedo, Goodman, Caballero, & Waldrop-Valverde, 2015), participants' responses to the items of the scale related to a simulated informed consent interview were significantly related to their overall health literacy.

Screening

Scales to measure health literacy can be used for a number of purposes. One person may be interested in understanding health literacy's relation to quality of life or risk of dying or health disparities, while another wants a quick and easy way to identify people who may need extra help in understanding a standard set of medication instructions included in a clinic's electronic health record. The first person may need a measure that assesses a broad range of content and may be able to use a scale that takes more than a few minutes to administer and score, while the second person is likely to want something shorter.

A person who wants to identify people who may have a problem understanding medication directions might be described as wanting a validated screening measure. How well screening measures identify people can be described with several indexes, the most important of which are the following. Since no test is perfect, these indexes give an idea of how confident someone can be about making a decision based on a test score.

Table 4-4. Characteristics of scale cutoff scores predicting low health literacy as reading level less than 8th grade

	Sensitivity	Specificity	Accuracy	PPV[a]	NPV[a]
HL40	0.79	0.66	0.72	0.64	0.81
Paper	0.79	0.64	0.71	0.62	0.81
Screener	0.70	0.70	0.71	0.76	0.63
TOFHLA	0.78	0.65	0.71	0.63	0.80

[a]PPV = positive predictive value; NPV = negative predictive value. Values are based on Youden index for all measures except screener which is based on a minimum PPV of 0.75.

Based on these values, you can choose a cutoff score that is appropriate to the purpose of your assessment.

Sensitivity. This is the number of persons who have a positive test divided by those who actually have a condition (for example, low health literacy). These are considered "true positives." Since almost no test can detect everyone with a problem or condition, this number is usually less than one. Many medical and psychological tests have sensitivity values in the range of 0.70 to 0.80.

Specificity. This is the proportion of people who don't have a condition who have a negative test. These are "true negatives." As with positive test values, few tests are 100% accurate. Many widely-used tests have specificity values in the range of 0.70 to 0.80.

Positive predictive value (PPV). This is how likely it is that someone with a *positive* test actually *has* the problem or condition, such as low health literacy. A PPV value of 0.80, for example, would mean that you

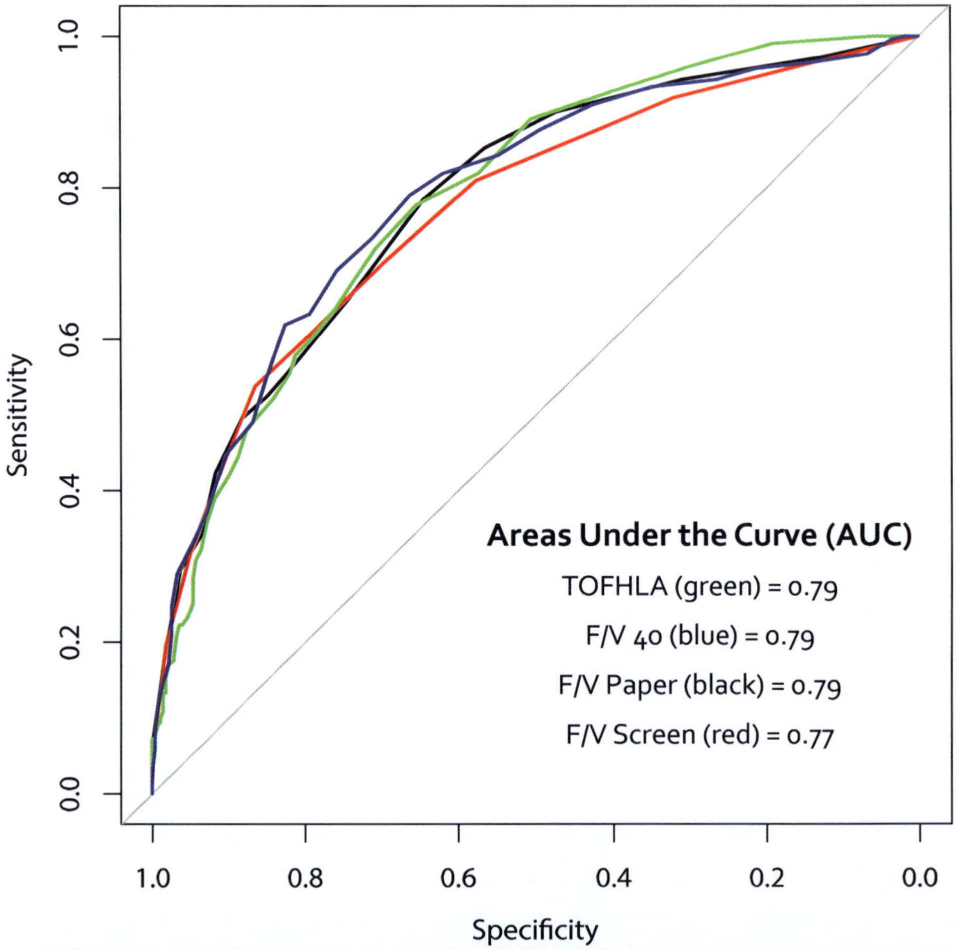

Figure 4-2. ROC Curves for TOFHLA Total Score, F/V 40-item general health literacy scale, F/V 20-item paper scale, and 10-item screening tool detecting persons with an 8th-grade or lower reading level

could be 80% sure that a person with a positive score actually has low health literacy.

Negative predictive value (NPV). This is how likely it is that someone with a *negative* test actually *doesn't* have the problem or condition–that is, probably has adequate health literacy.

Accuracy. Accuracy is the total number of correct identified individuals (whether they are correctly considered to have or not have the condition) divided by the total number of persons assessed.

These indexes depend on the cutoff score used, so it's possible to have different cutoff scores depending on whether you want a highly sensitive or highly specific test. PPV and NPV also depend on how common the condition (like low health literacy) is in the group of persons tested. In the tables for F/V scales provided here, a prevalence of low health literacy of 50% is assumed based on the overall estimate o the prevalence of health literacy reported in a review study (Paasche-Orlow, Parker, Gazmararian, Nielsen-Bohlman, & Rudd, 2005).

Deciding on cutoff scores

If someone wants to be sure of identifying everyone with low health literacy, even if it means some people might be identified as having low health literacy even though they don't, a cutoff score with a high sensitivity would be used. If this is done, almost everyone who might need help will be identified, but some people who don't need help would also be included.

One common strategy for deciding on cutoff scores is to employ a technique called receiver operating curve (ROC) analysis. Calculation of sensitivities and specificities for a range of cutoffs provides data to plot various combinations of sensitivity and specificity in a curve (Figure 4-2). Figure 4-2 shows ROC curves for the TOFHLA total score, the F/V 40-item health literacy scale, the 20-item paper and pencil scale, and the F/V 10-item screening tool. The criterion used in these analyses was whether someone had a Woodcock-Johnson or Woodcock-Muñoz Passage Comprehension scores at or below the 8th grade level (suggesting less than adequate level of health literacy). The figure suggests that all the measures perform about equally well in identifying people with low levels of reading skill. Similar curves were obtained using the criterion of less than 4th grade reading level.

The performance of a measure in ROC analysis can also be characterized in part based on the area under the curve (AUC) associated with its ROC curve. The areas under the curve were: TOFHLA total score = 0.79; F/V HL40 = 0.79; F/V 20 item paper and pencil scale = 0.79; F/V 10 item screening tool = 0.77. None of these values was significantly different from any of the others (Delong's test of correlated ROC curves; all *ps* > 0.05) although the test of the difference between the F/V 20-item paper and pencil scale and 10-item screening tool approached significance ($z = 1.78$, $p = 0.08$). At least for the criterion of detecting a person who may have less than 8th grade reading level, all the measures perform in a similar fashion, with the F/V scales performing as well as the longer TOFHLA.

People are sometimes surprised to find out that a test result doesn't mean something with certainty. This is true not only in the realm of health literacy tests, but many other tests as well. For example, reported sensitivities and specificities for the TOFHLA and the Newest Vital Sign are in the range of 0.70 to 0.75 (Osborn et al., 2007; Weiss et al., 2005). Combined with internal reliabilities in the same range (Cronbach's alpha), any person's score on these measures should be interpreted cautiously, probably in the context of the person's education and the complexity of the health literacy challenge they are presented in real life.

Patterns of health literacy

If we want a measure of health literacy to identify those who have a problem understanding health information, it is necessary to decide on on a criterion to define what "low health literacy" means. For a number of health literacy measures such as the S-TOFHLA and the NVS, low health literacy is defined based on cutoff scores from the TOFHLA development sample. In that study, the TOFHLA was administered to a large number of people; those who scored below the average were considered to have "Inadequate" health literacy, while those with other scores were considered as having either "Marginal" or "Adequate" health literacy. A problem with that approach that the definition of low health literacy was defined was not related to an external criterion–scores on the TOFHLA, S-TOFHLA,

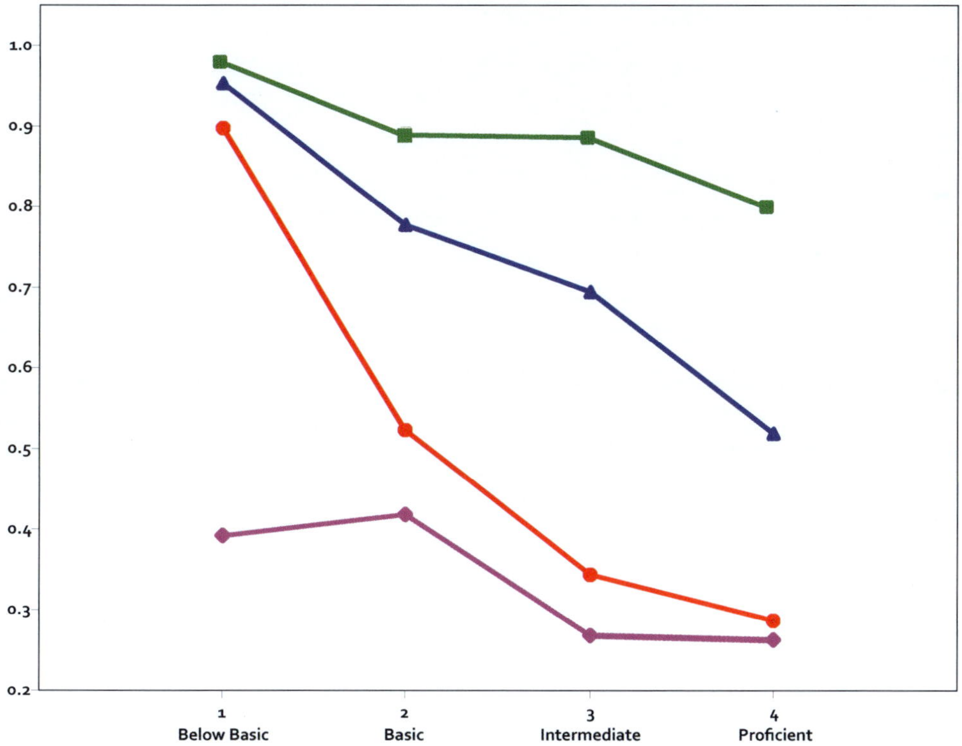

Figure 4-3. Median proportion of items from each category answered correctly by individuals in each group. Group: Purple = Low Health Literacy; Red = Basic; Blue = Averagee; Green = Proficient

NVS, and other measures keyed to the TOFHLA categories may not agree with other measures. As was discussed in Chapter 3 (section titled Distribution of Scores), in many studies a very large number of people score in the Adequate range on the TOFHLA, making its usefulness questionable. In defining low health literacy in F/V, we therefore chose to examine alternative ways to operationally define "low health literacy."

In defining low health literacy, we looked at several different ways of deciding who has adequate or low health literacy. Since all participants completed the TOFHLA, it was possible to decide who had low health literacy based on the traditional cutoff scores used for that measure. F/V participants also completed an individually-administered and well standardized and normed measure of reading comprehension. While general reading comprehension isn't the same thing health literacy, it is likely that persons with low levels of academic reading skills (below the 8th grade level, for example) might have difficulties in the skills component of the ASK model (see Chapter Two). We thus also explored the extent to which FLIGHT/VIDAS scales can identify individuals who scored below the 8th grade level on this general reading comprehension measure. Finally, we asked participants questions about their level of difficulty in understanding written health information. Those who reported having difficulty in understanding written health information were considered as well. As demonstrated in this chapter, the F/V scales perform well in identfying persons in groups based on these criteria.

In addition, we chose to pursue a more qualitative description of indi-

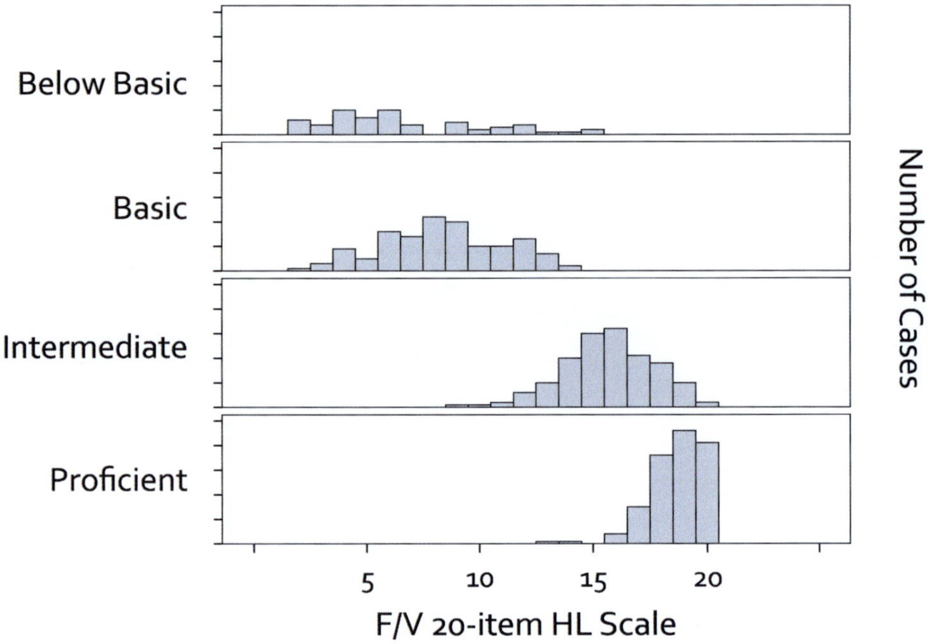

Figure 4-4. Distribution to F/V scores in health literacy proficiency groups.

viudals' levels of health literacy based on the levels developed for the National Assessment of Adult Literacy (Kutner et al. 2006). These groupings were developed based on an analysis of the tasks required in answering the items on that measure. Persons with Below Basic skills are able to complete items with ". . .no more than the most simple and concrete literacy skills" (Kutner et al. 2006, p. 5). Persons with Basic skills have the skills "necessary to perform simple and everyday . . .activities" while those with Intermediate skills can ". . . perform moderately challenging . . .activities" (p. 5). Finally, those with Proficient skills can complete ". . .more complex and challenging . . .activities" (p. 5).

In examining how we mightprovide a cleare qualitative description of our participants' levels of health literacy, the items from F/V that could be readily categorized according to the NAAL criteria. We created separate scores for each particpant based on the proportion of items answered correctly in the groups that reflect different tasks demands. These scores were then used in latent class analysis to create groups of persons with qualitatively different patterns of health literacy (Ownby, Acevedo, Waldrop-Valverde, manuscript in preparation). We found distinct groups of individuals based on their performance on the different types of health literacy questions (Figure 4-3).

We found that some persons had difficulty with nearly all items across types of questions, but were more likely to answer the questions in the Below Basic and Basic groups (purple line in the figure). This group, which had difficulty with even basic and straightforward health literacy tasks, is referred to as having Low Health Literacy as they were only able to complete a portion of the simplest tasks in F/V. Of these individuals, 86% correctly answered a question about the number of persons missing in a picture but only 32% correctly answered a question that required a straightforward application of information from a table of body mass index values. Only 45% could correctly answer a question involving mental calculation related to grams of carbohydrate when given information in a simple table. These individuals' performance on an academic reading measure (Woodcock-Johnson or Woodcock-Muñoz Passage Comprehension test) was at the late primary grade level (4th-6th grades), and it appears likely that they would have difficulty with any but the simplest written instructions about managing their health.

A second group performed fairly well on the Below Basic group of questions and moderately well on the Basic items, but less well on Intermediate and Proficient questions (red line). These persons can be characterized as having Basic health literacy. Individuals in the Basic group were likely to answer the questions ranked as below basic but were less likely to answer more complex questions even when they required extraction of single pieces of data from a table or simple but several stage arithmetic calculations (such as calculating the grams of fat even from several food sources). These individuals' performance on an academic reading measure was at the late primary grade level (about 6th grade).

A third group did well on items in the Below Basic, Basic, and Intermediate groups of items but not on the Proficient items. These individuals can be characterized as having Average health literacy (blue line). Individuals in the Average group could perform tasks of moderate complexity, such as extracting relevant information from a prose paragraph or completing an arithmetic calculation that involved several steps. Their performance on the academic reading measure was at about the 8th grade level.

Finally, a fourth group performed well on all groups of items and are clearly Proficient (green line). Individuals in the Proficient group were consistently able to extract and use information from complex prose or document sources, and could assess probability even in a complex scenario involving competing risks of treatment outcomes and side effects. This group's performance on the academic reading measure was at the 12th grade level.In examining each group's performances, it became evident that the health literacy of members of the groups could be described in terms of the kind of health literacy tasks the group's members could and could not perform.

Summary

Overall, results of assessments of F/V reliability and validity show that it has adequate reliability and validity for use as an assessment of health literacy. It is particularly noteworthy that the F/V 20 item scale is shorter than the full-length TOFHLA but performs as well with respect to identifying persons with low levels of literacy. Critically important is the wide range of difficulty in F/V scores, eliminating the problem of ceiling effects that plagues most other measures of health literacy.

5 Using FLIGHT/ VIDAS

As explained in previous chapters, the extensive item development process completed in the F/V project allowed us to identify a number of scales that can be used for different purposes (e.g., diagnostic assessment or screening) and to assess different aspects of health literacy (prose and document, numeracy, listening, conceptual health knowledge). If you're interested in using F/V, this chapter should help you decide which scale is best for your purpose.

The F/V scales can be administered in one of two ways (see Table 5-1, next page). Computer administration requires a tablet or desktop computer and an Internet connection. Paper and pencil administration requires this manual a booklet of test materials, and an answer sheet (see the F/V website at www.flightvidas.org for information about how to obtain these materials). Portions of questions should be read aloud to the person assessed because this was the way the questions were presented to people in the original validation study.

In our experience, most people will want to use a measure of health literacy for one of the following reasons:

Screening for low health literacy

If this is what you want to do, use the 10-item paper and pencil screener. This will take 10-15 minutes, and you can score it as you go along. The answer sheet has a table to let you know how the person performed on the

Table 5-1. Available F/V scales

Scale	Access	Items	Time	Purpose
Paper	Paper	20	15-20	Assess general health literacy
Screen	Paper	10	10-12	Screen for low health literacy
HL40	Computer	40	20-30	Diagnostic assessment of prose and document health literacy
NUM	Computer	29	20-30	Diagnostic assessment of numeracy skills
LIS	Computer	13	15	Assess listening skills in simulated clinical encounter, patient education, and research settings

measure in relation to other in their age group (see Tables 5–4 and 5–5). The normative tables provide T scores that have an average fo 50 and a standard deviation of 10. See Table A-1 in Appendix IV for information on interpreting T scores if you're not familiar with this type of score.

The 10-item screener is also available for computer administration. You can find out how to access the computer version on the F/V website at www.fligthvidas.org. The computer version will generate a score and interpretation, but requires a computer or tablet and an Internet connection.

Normative data for the screening tool is available in the form of T scores (see Table 5-4 and 5-5). The scores are based on the average performance of our participants in each age group so that a person's performance on the scale can be understood in relation to their age. It's important to note

Table 5-2. T Score Equivalents of Raw Scores on the English 20-item HL Scale

Raw Score	18-29	30-39	40-49	50-59	60-69	70 and older
1	2	14	26	18	22	22
2	5	17	28	20	25	24
3	8	19	30	23	27	26
4	11	21	32	25	29	28
5	14	24	34	27	31	30
6	17	26	36	30	33	32
7	21	28	37	32	35	34
8	24	31	39	34	37	36
9	27	33	41	37	39	39
10	30	35	43	39	41	41
11	33	38	45	42	44	43
12	36	40	47	44	46	45
13	39	42	49	46	48	47
14	42	45	51	49	50	49
15	45	47	53	51	52	51
16	48	49	55	53	54	53
17	51	52	57	56	56	55
18	54	54	58	58	58	57
19	57	56	60	60	60	59
20	60	59	62	63	63	61

that these scores are not adjusted for level of education. This means that when interpreting the score should also take into account someone's level of education. These scores can help you understand how a person's level of health literacy compares to other people in the same age group. If you are only interested in knowing whether the person has low, basic, or higher health literacy, you should use the cutoff scores on the answer sheet.

Assessing health literacy

You may be interested in doing a more in-depth assessment of a person's health literacy in a way that takes no more than 20-30 minutes. For this purpose, use the 20-item health literacy scale. It will give you information about the person's overall level of health literacy, a more precise estimate of the person's needs with respect to written health communications, and examination of specific items will give you insight into the person's strengths and weaknesses in understanding health information. This scale includes a number of items that require numeracy skills.

Normative data is available for this scale, too (see Tables 5-2 and 5-3). These data provide T scores that will help you understand how well a person scores on the test compared to other people in their age group.

This scale is available in a paper and pencil version. As with the screener, the paper and pencil version should be administered according to the instructions in the test booklet, with portions of the questions read aloud to the person assessed. This scale is also available for computer administration. You can also find out how to access this scale on our website at www.fligthvidas.org. The computer version will generate a score and interpretation, but requires a computer or tablet and an Internet connection.

Researching health literacy

The F/V project developed data on a longer 40-item general health literacy scale as well as the numeracy (NUM), Listening (LIS), and conceptual health knowledge (FACT) scales described in Chapter 3. Each of these

Table 5-3. T Score Equivalents of Raw Scores on the Spanish 20-item HL Scale

Raw Score	18-29	30-39	40-49	50-59	60-69	70 and older
1	12	13	21	27	33	35
2	15	16	23	29	35	37
3	17	18	25	31	37	40
4	20	21	28	33	39	42
5	23	23	30	35	41	44
6	25	26	32	37	43	47
7	28	28	34	39	45	49
8	31	31	36	40	47	52
9	33	33	39	42	49	54
10	36	36	41	44	51	56
11	39	38	43	46	53	59
12	41	41	45	48	55	61
13	44	43	47	50	57	64
14	46	46	50	52	59	66
15	49	48	52	54	61	68
16	52	50	54	56	63	71
17	54	53	56	58	65	73
18	57	55	58	60	67	76
19	60	58	61	62	69	78
20	62	60	63	64	71	80

scales is currently only available for computer administration, although a paper and pencil version of the FACT scale is currently being developed. For information on how to access and use these scales, please contact us via the F/V website at www.flightvidas.org.

Using F/V items to study something else

Because of the diverse content and formats of the F/V items, several interested researchers have used them to develop scales to evaluate other aspects of health literacy for specific purposes. One of the F/V team, Josh Caballero, PharmD, used F/V items to create a scale relevant to pharmacist counseling on medication management. Another person is working with us in creating a scale that can assess aspects of health literacy relevant to pediatrics. This manual and the F/V website will be updated as more information about these projects becomes available.

Summary

This chapter has briefly described how to use F/V for the most common purposes we have encountered. Please contact us for additional information about using F/V or for any questions. The most up to date information on F/V will always be available at www.flightvidas.org.

Table 5-4. T Score Equivalents of Raw Scores on the English 10-item Screening Tool

Raw Score	18-29	30-39	40-49	50-59	60-69	70 and older
1	10	16	30	25	26	26
2	15	21	33	29	30	29
3	21	26	37	33	34	33
4	26	30	40	37	38	37
5	32	35	44	41	42	41
6	37	39	47	45	45	45
7	43	44	51	49	49	49
8	48	49	55	52	53	52
9	53	53	58	56	57	56
10	59	58	62	60	61	60

Table 5-5. T Score Equivalents of Raw Scores on the Spanish 10-item Screening Tool

Raw Score	18-29	30-39	40-49	50-59	60-69	70 and older
1	11	18	20	30	34	39
2	16	23	24	33	38	43
3	22	27	29	37	42	47
4	27	32	33	40	46	52
5	33	36	38	44	50	56
6	38	40	42	47	54	60
7	44	45	47	51	58	64
8	49	49	52	54	62	68
9	55	54	56	58	66	73
10	61	58	61	61	70	77

References

Acevedo, A., Krueger, K. R., Navarro, E., Ortiz, F., Manly, J. J., Padilla-Velez, M. M. et al. (2009). The Spanish translation and adaptation of the Uniform Data Set of the National Institute on Aging Alzheimer's Disease Centers. *Alzheimer Disease and Associated Disorders*, 23, 102-109.

Ackerman, P. L., Beier, M. E., & Bowen, K. R. (2000). Explorations of crystallized intelligence: Completion tests, cloze tests, and knowledge. *Learning and Individual Differences*, 12, 105-121.

Ackerman, P. L. & Cianciolo, A. T. (2000). Cognitive, perceptual-speed, and psychomotor determinants of individual differences during skill acquisition. *Journal of Experimental Psycholofy: Applied*, 6, 259-290.

Aguirre, A. C., Ebrahim, N., & Shea, J. A. (2005). Performance of the English and Spanish S-TOFHLA among publicly insured Medicaid and Medicare patients. *Patient Education and Counseling*, 56, 332-339.

Baker, D. W. (2006). The meaning and the measure of health literacy. *Journal of General Internal Medicine*, 21, 878-883.

Baker, D. W., Gazmararian, J. A., Sudano, J., Patterson, M., Parker, R. M., & Williams, M. V. (2002). Health literacy and performance on the Mini-Mental State Examination. *Aging and Mental Health*, 6, 22-29.

Baker, D. W., Wolf, M. S., Feinglass, J., & Thompson, J. A. (2008). Health literacy, cognitive abilities, and mortality among elderly persons. *Journal of General Internal Medicine*, 23, 723-726.

Bass, P. F., III, Wilson, J. F., & Griffith, C. H. (2003). A shortened instrument for literacy screening. *Journal of General Internal Medicine*, 18, 1036-1038.

Berkman, N. D., Sheridan, S. L., Donahue, K. E., Halpern, D. J., & Crotty, K. (2011). Low health literacy and health outcomes: an updated systematic review. *Annals of Internal Medicine*, 155, 97-107.

Charness, N. & Tuffiash, M. (2008). The role of expertise research and human factors in capturing, explaining, and producing superior performance. *Human Factors*, 50, 427-432.

Chesser, A. K., Keene Woods, N., Wipperman, J., Wilson, R., & Dong, F. (2014). Health literacy assessment of the STOFHLA: Paper versus electronic administration continuation study. *Health Education & Behavior*, 41, 19-24.

Chew, L. D., Bradley, K. A., & Boyko, E. J. (2004). Brief questions to identify patients with inadequate health literacy. *Family Medicine*, 36, 588-594.

Chin, J., Morrow, D. G., Stine-Morrow, E. A., Conner-Garcia, T., Graumlich, J. F., & Murray, M. D. (2011). The process-knowledge model of health literacy: evidence from a componential analysis of two commonly used measures. *Journal of Health Communication*, 16 Suppl 3, 222-241.

Deary, I. J., Pattie, A., & Starr, J. M. (2013). The stability of intelligence from age 11 to age 90 years: the Lothian birth cohort of 1921. *Psychological Science*, 24, 2361-2368.

Department of Health and Human Services (2011). *Healthy people 2020: Topics and objectives.* Washington DC: Department of Health and Human Services. Available at http://healthypeople.gov/2020/topicsobjectives2020/pdfs/HP2020objectives.pdf. Accessed August 1, 2011.

DeVellis, R. F. (2006). Classical test theory. *Medical Care*, 44, S50-S59.

Embretson, S. E. & Reise, S. P. (2000). *Item response theory for psychologists.* Mahwah, NJ: Lawrence Erlbaum.

Federman, A. D., Sano, M., Wolf, M. S., Siu, A. L., & Halm, E. A. (2009). Health literacy and cognitive performance in older adults. *Journal of the American Geriatrics Society*, 57, 1475-1480.

Folstein, M. F., Folstein, S. E., & McHugh, P. R. (1975). "Mini-mental state." A practical method for grading the cognitive state of patients for the clinician. *Journal of Psychiatry Research*, 12, 189-198.

Gazmararian, J. A., Williams, M. V., Peel, J., & Baker, D. W. (2003). Health literacy and knowledge of chronic disease. *Patient Education and Counseling*, 51, 267-275.

Griffin, J. M., Partin, M. R., Noorbaloochi, S., Grill, J. P., Saha, S., Snyder, A. et al. (2010). Variation in estimates of limited health literacy by assessment instruments and non-response bias. *Journal of General Internal Medicine*, 25, 675-681.

Gulliksen, H. (1950). *Theory of mental tests*. New York: Wiley.

Gwaltney, C. J., Shields, A. L., & Shiffman, S. (2008). Equivalence of electronic and paper-and-pencil administration of patient-reported outcome measures: a meta-analytic review. *Value in Health*, 11, 322-333.

Haun, J., Luther, S., Dodd, V., & Donaldson, P. (2012). Measurement variation across health literacy assessments: implications for assessment selection in research and practice. *Journal of Health Communication*, 17 Suppl 3, 141-159.

Hicks, G., Barragan, M., Franco-Paredes, C., Williams, M. V., & Del, R. C. (2006). Health literacy is a predictor of HIV/AIDS knowledge. *Family Medicine*, 38, 717-723.

Horn, J. L. & Cattell, R. B. (1966). Refinement and test of the theory of fluid and crystallized general intelligences. *Journal of Educational Psychology*, 57, 253-270.

Jerant, A., Sohler, N., Fiscella, K., Franks, B., & Franks, P. (2011). Tailored interactive multimedia computer programs to reduce health disparities: opportunities and challenges. *Patient Education and Counseling*, 85, 323-330.

Jordan, J. E., Osborne, R. H., & Buchbinder, R. (2011). Critical appraisal of health literacy indices revealed variable underlying constructs, narrow content and psychometric weaknesses. *Journal of Clinical Epidemiology*, 64, 366-379.

Kirsch, I. (2001). *The International Adult Literacy Survey (IALS): Understanding what was measured.* Princeton, NJ: Educational Testing Service.

Kirsch, I. S., Jungeblut, A., Jenkins, L., & Kolstad, A. (2002). *Adult literacy in America: A first look at the findings of the National Adult Literacy Survey.* Washington DC: National Center for Educational Statistics.

Kruidenier, J. R., MacArthur, C. A., & Wrigley, H. S. (2010). *Adult education literacy instruction: A review of the research.* Washington, DC: National Institute for Literacy.

Kutner, M., Greenberg, E., Jin, Y., & Paulsen, C. (2006). *The health literacy of America's adults: Results from the 2003 National Asessment of Adult Literacy (NCES 2006-483).* Washington, DC: US Department of Education, National Center for Educational Statistics.

Lee, S. Y., Bender, D. E., Ruiz, R. E., & Cho, Y. I. (2006). Development of an easy-to-use Spanish health literacy test. *Health Services Research*, 41, 1392-1412.

Levinthal, B. R., Morrow, D. G., Tu, W., Wu, J., & Murray, M. D. (2008). Cognition and health literacy in patients with hypertension. *Journal of General Internal Medicine*, 23, 1172-1176.

Lord, F. M. & Novick, M. R. (1968). *Statistical theories of mental test scores*. Boston, MA: Addison-Wesley.

Lustria, M. L., Noar, S. M., Cortese, J., Van Stee, S. K., Glueckauf, R. L., & Lee, J. (2013). A meta-analysis of web-delivered tailored health behavior change interventions. *Journal of Health Communication*, 18, 1039-1069.

Marin, G., Sabogal, F., Marin, B. V., Otero-Sabogal, R., & Perez-Stable, E. J. (1987). Development of a short acculturation scale for Hispanics. *Hispanic Journal of Behavioral Sciences*, 9, 183-205.

Meyer, J. P. (2014). *Applied measurement with jMetrik.* New York: Routledge.

Millsap, C. M. (2000). *Comparison of computer testing versus traditional paper and pencil testing* (Doctoral Dissertation). University of North Texas.

Mottus, R., Johnson, W., Murray, C., Wolf, M. S., Starr, J. M., & Deary, I. J. (2014). Towards understanding the links between health literacy and physical health. *Health Psychology*, 33, 164-173.

Murphy, P. W., Davis, T. C., Long, S. W., Jackson, R. H., & Decker, B. C. (1993). Rapid Estimate of Adult Literacy in Medicine (REALM): A quick reading test for patients. *Journal of Reading*, 37, 124-130.

Muthén, L. K. & Muthén, B. O. (2012). *Mplus user's guide (7th ed.)*. Los Angeles: Muthén & Muthén.

Nielsen-Bohlman, L., Panzer, A. M., & Kindig, D. A. (2004). *Health literacy: A prescription to end confusion.* Washington DC: National Academies Press.

Noar, S. M., Benac, C. N., & Harris, M. S. (2007). Does tailoring matter? Meta-analytic review of tailored print health behavior change interventions. *Psychological Bulletin*, 133, 673-693.

Orlando, M. (2004). Critical issues to address when applying item response theory (IRT) models. Paper presented at the conference Advances in Health Outcomes Measurement: Exploring the Current State and the Future of Item Response Theory, Item Banks, and Computer-Adaptive Testing, Bethesda, MD, June.

Osborn, C. Y., Cavanaugh, K., Wallston, K. A., Kripalani, S., Elasy, T. A., Rothman, R. L. et al. (2011). Health literacy explains racial disparities in diabetes medication adherence. *Journal of Health Communication*, 16 Suppl 3, 268-278.

Osborn, C. Y., Weiss, B. D., Davis, T. C., Skripkauskas, S., Rodrigue, C., Bass, P. F. et al. (2007). Measuring adult literacy in health care: Performance of the Newest Vital Sign. *American Journal of Health Behavior*, 31 Suppl 1, S36-S46.

Ownby, R. L., Acevedo, A., Goodman, K., Caballero, J., & Waldrop-Valverde, D. (2015). Health literacy predicts participant understanding of orally-presented informed consent information. *Clinical Research and Trials*, 1, 15-19.

Ownby, R. L., Acevedo, A., Jacobs, R. J., Caballero, J., & Waldrop-Valverde, D. (2014a). Negative and positive beliefs related to mood and health. A*American Journal of Health Behavior*, 38, 586-597.

Ownby, R. L., Acevedo, A., Jacobs, R. J., Caballero, J., & Waldrop-Valverde, D. (2014b). Quality of life, health status, and health service utilization related to a new measure of health literacy: FLIGHT/VIDAS. *Patient Education and Counseling*, 94, 404-410.

Ownby, R. L., Acevedo, A., Waldrop-Valverde, D., & Jacobs, R. J. (2014). Is the cloze procedure appropriate to evaluate health literacy in older individuals? Age effects in the test of functional health literacy in adults. *Journal of Aging Research*, 2014, 194635.

Ownby, R. L., Acevedo, A., Waldrop-Valverde, D., Jacobs, R. J., & Caballero, J. (2013). A new computer-administered measure of health literacy: Validity and relation to quality of life in Spanish and English speakers. Paper presented at the International Conference on Communication in Healthcare, Montreal, October.

Ownby, R. L., Acevedo, A., Waldrop-Valverde, D., Jacobs, R. J., & Caballero, J. (2014). Abilities, skills and knowledge in measures of health literacy. *Patient Education and Counseling*, 95, 211-217.

Ownby, R. L., Acevedo, A., Waldrop-Valverde, D., Jacobs, R. J., Homs, A. M., Czaja, S. J. et al. (2013). Development and initial validation of a computer-administered health literacy assessment in Spanish and English: FLIGHT/VIDAS. *Patient Related Outcome Measures*, 4, 1-15.

Ownby, R. L., Hertzog, C., & Czaja, S. J. (2012). Tailored information and automated reminding to improve medication adherence in Spanish- and English-speaking elders treated for memory impairment. *Clinical Gerontologist*, 35, 221-238.

Ownby, R. L. & Waldrop-Valverde, D. (2009). Health literacy is related to problem solving. Paper presented at the Health Literacy Research Conference. Washington DC, October..

Ownby, R. L. & Waldrop-Valverde, D. (2013). Differential item functioning related to age in the Reading subtest of the Test of Functional Health Literacy in Adults. *Journal of Aging Research*, 2013, 1-6.

Ownby, R. L., Waldrop-Valverde, D., Caballero, J., & Jacobs, R. J. (2012). Baseline medication adherence and response to an electronically delivered health literacy intervention targeting adherence. *Neurobehavioral HIV Medicine*, 4, 113-121.

Ownby, R. L., Waldrop-Valverde, D., Hardigan, P., Caballero, J., Jacobs, R., & Acevedo, A. (2013). Development and validation of a brief computer-administered HIV-related health literacy scale (HIV-HL). *AIDS & Behavior*, 17, 710-718.

Paasche-Orlow, M. K., Parker, R. M., Gazmararian, J. A., Nielsen-Bohlman, L. T., & Rudd, R. R. (2005). The prevalence of limited health literacy. *Journal of General Internal Medicine*, 20, 175-184.

Paasche-Orlow, M. K. & Wolf, M. S. (2007). The causal pathways linking health literacy to health outcomes. *American Journal of Health Behavior*, 31 Suppl 1, S19-S26.

Parker, R. M., Baker, D. W., Williams, M. V., & Nurss, J. R. (1995). The Test of Functional Health Literacy in Adults: A new instrument for measuring patients' literacy skills. *Journal of General Internal Medicine*, 10, 537-541.

Pleasant, A., McKinney, J., & Rikard, R. V. (2011). Health literacy measurement: a proposed research agenda. *Journal of Health Communication*, 16 Suppl 3, 11-21.

Ramirez-Zohfeld, V., Rademaker, A. W., Dolan, N. C., Ferreira, M. R., Eder, M. M., Liu, D. et al. (2015). Comparing the performance of the S-TOFHLA and NVS among and between English and Spanish speakers. J*Journal of Health Communication*, Online July 15, 2015, 1-7.

Reingold, E. M., Charness, N., Pomplun, M., & Stampe, D. M. (2001). Visual span in expert chess players: evidence from eye movements. *Psychological Science*, 12, 48-55.

Roring, R. W. & Charness, N. (2007). A multilevel model analysis of expertise in chess across the life span. *Psychology and Aging*, 22, 291-299.

Rothman, R. L., Malone, R., Bryant, B., Wolfe, C., Padgett, P., Dewalt, D. A. et al. (2005). The Spoken Knowledge in Low Literacy in Diabetes scale: a diabetes knowledge scale for vulnerable patients. *Diabetes Education*, 31, 215-224.

Schwartz, K. L., Bartoces, M., Campbell-Voytal, K., West, P., Monsur, J., Sartor, A. et al. (2013). Estimating health literacy in family medicine clinics in metropolitan Detroit: a MetroNet study. *Journal of the American Board of Family Medicine*, 26, 566-570.

Sorensen, K., Van den Broucke, S., Pelikan, J., Fullam, J., Doyle, G., Slonska, Z. et al. (2013). Measuring health literacy in populations: illuminating the design and development process of the European Health Literacy Survey Questionnaire (HLS-EU-Q). *BMC Public Health*, 13, 948.

The Centre for Health Literacy. (2011). The Calgary Charter on health literacy. Montréal, The Centre for Health Literacy. Online at: http://www.centreforliteracy.qc.ca/sites/default/files/CFL_Calgary_Charter_2011.pdf.

Wechsler, D. (1944). *The measurement of adult intelligence, 3rd ed.* Baltimore: Williams & Wilkins.

Wechsler, D. (1958). *The measurement and appraisal of adult intelligence, 4th ed.* Baltimore: Williams & Wilkins.

Weiss, B. D., Mays, M. Z., Martz, W., Castro, K. M., Dewalt, D. A., Pignone, M. P. et al. (2005). Quick assessment of literacy in primary care: The Newest Vital Sign. *Annals of Family Medicine*, 3, 514-522.

Wingersky, M. S. & Lord, F. M. (1984). An investigation of methods for reducing sampling error in certain IRT procedures. *Applied Psychological Measurement*, 8, 347-364.

Wolf, M. S., Curtis, L. M., Wilson, E. A., Revell, W., Waite, K. R., Smith, S. G. et al. (2012). Literacy, cognitive function, and health: Results of the LitCog study. *Journal of General Internal Medicine*, 27, 1300-1307.

Woodcock, R. W., McGrew, K. S., & Mather, N. (2007). *Woodcock-Johnson III Normative Update.* Rolling Meadows, IL: Riverside.

Woodcock, R. W., Muñoz-Sandoval, A. F., McGrew, K. S., & Mather, N. (2007). *Batería III Woodcock-Muñoz.* Rolling Meadows, IL: Riverside.

Yost, K. J., Dewalt, D. A., Lindquist, L. A., & Hahn, E. A. (2013). The association between health literacy and indicators of cognitive impairment in a diverse sample of primary care patients. *Patient Education and Counseling*, 93, 319-326.

I Development

NOTE: This is the final version of a published manuscript. The definitive edition appears on the website of *Patient Related Outcome Measures* at https://www.dovepress.com/patient-related-outcome-measures-journal

Development and Initial Validation of a Computer-Administered Health Literacy Assessment in Spanish and English: FLIGHT/VIDAS

Raymond L Ownby(1)

Amarilis Acevedo(2)

Drenna Waldrop-Valverde(3)

Robin J. Jacobs(1)

Joshua Caballero(4)

Rosemary Davenport(1)

Ana-Maria Homs(1)

Sara J. Czaja(5)

David Loewenstein(5)

(1) Department of Psychiatry and Behavioral Medicine, Nova Southeastern University, Fort Lauderdale, FL

(2) Center for Psychological Studies, Nova Southeastern University, Fort Lauderdale, FL

(3) Nell Hodgson Woodruff School of Nursing, Emory University, Atlan-

ta, GA

(4) College of Pharmacy, Department of Pharmacy Practice, Nova Southeastern University, Fort Lauderdale, FL

(5) University of Miami Miller School of Medicine, Miami, FL

Correspondence to: Dr. Ownby, Room 1477, 3200 South University Drive, Fort Lauderdale FL 33314. E-mail: ro71@nova.edu; Voice: +1-954-262-1481.

Supported by grant R01HL096578 from the National Heart, Lung, and Blood Institute to Dr. Ownby.

ABSTRACT

Current measures of health literacy have been criticized on a number of grounds, including a limited range of content, development on small and atypical patient groups, and poor psychometric characteristics. In this paper we report the development and preliminary validation of a new computer-administered and scored health literacy measure addressing these limitations. Items reflect a wide range of content related to health promotion and maintenance as well as care for diseases. The development process has focused on creating a measure that will be useful in both Spanish and English while not requiring substantial time for clinician training and individual administration and scoring. Items incorporate several formats including questions based on brief videos that allow for assessment of listening comprehension and skills related to obtaining information on the Internet. In this paper we report interim analyses detailing the initial development and pilot testing of the items (phase 1 of the project) in groups of Spanish and English speakers. We then describe phase 2 that includes a second round of testing the items in new groups of Spanish and English speakers and evaluation of the new measure's reliability and validity in relation to other measures. Data are presented that show that four scales (general health literacy, numeracy, conceptual knowledge, and listening comprehension) developed through a process of item and factor analyses have significant relations to existing measures of health literacy.

RUNNING HEAD: FLIGHT/VIDAS

KEYWORDS: Health literacy, cognition, disparities, item response theory

Health literacy, defined as an individual's ability to obtain health-related information and use it to make decisions,1 is increasingly recognized as an important factor in patient health. Several reviews show that individuals' health literacy is related to their health status, function, and use of services2;3 and it has even been related to increased risk of mortality.4;5 The existence of effective interventions to improve health literacy6;7 highlights the possibility that improving it may be a strategy for improving health outcomes and addressing race- and ethnicity-related health disparities.8;9

Commonly used measures of health literacy include the Test of Functional Health Literacy in Adults, or TOFHLA,10 the Rapid Estimate of Adult Literacy in Medicine, or REALM,11 and the Newest Vital Sign.12 Each measure has strengths and weaknesses. The TOFHLA, for example, assesses a patients' ability to understand what they read as well as their numeracy skills. A limitation of the TOFHLA, however, is the requirement that the clinician administering it be trained and the time required for the clinician to individually administer and score it, typically at least 30 minutes. The time required for administration thus limits its use in clinical and research settings. .A shorter version, the S-TOFHLA, is available13 but suffers from ceiling effects (many people achieve high scores) that limit its use in research since a limited range of scores affects the ability to detect its relations to other variables.

The REALM also must be administered, scored and interpreted by a trained clinician. This measure only assesses health literacy as patients' ability to correctly pronounce a series of health related words (e.g., anatomical terms and the names of diseases and condition) and thus does not directly assess their ability to understand what they read. The REALM does not assess numeracy skills, consistently shown to be an important aspect of health literacy. The Newest Vital Sign only assesses patients' comprehension of a single food label, and thus only taps a very narrow range of skills. It may have limited use except perhaps for the purpose of detecting whether a patient has poor reading comprehension skills.

Baker noted the limitations of existing measures of health literacy some time ago14 and problems encountered in assessing it are summarized more recently by Pleasant and McKinney15 and in an empirical review by Jordan et al.16 Existing measures have been criticized for assessing a limited set of skills and for their development using patients drawn from single racial, ethnic, age, or socioeconomic groups. Other criticisms have noted the limited content and face validity of the measures and limited demonstrations of the measures' construct validity.16 Further, although both Spanish and English versions of several measures are available, they were not developed using psychometric procedures that establish their equivalence across languages making comparisons difficult.

An issue limiting the usefulness of the TOFHLA is the response format it uses in evaluating reading comprehension. The TOFHLA uses the cloze procedure17 to assess reading comprehension. In this approach, comprehension is tested by asking the person assessed to supply a word missing in a sentence (e.g., "The sky is _____"). This approach may create items that are differentially more difficult for older persons. Cloze procedure performance has been related to information processing speed and verbal fluency, reduced in older persons,18 and data presented in a paper currently submitted for publication from our group suggest the presence of differential item functioning (DIF) on a significant number of items from the reading comprehension subtest of the TOFHLA for people over 50. Item DIF occurs when individuals from different groups such as men or women or racial groups, who have the same level of ability, have different probabilities of answering an item correctly. The empirical finding of this kind of difference is usually interpreted as evidence that some factor besides the person's actual ability affects their performance, perhaps cultural, linguistic, or some other bias.[19] The finding of age-related DIF on the TOFHLA reading comprehension subtest suggests that other item formats (e.g., multiple choice questions) may be more appropriate for use in assessing health literacy in older persons.

Almost all existing paper-and-pencil measures require hand scoring, making them time- and effort-intensive. Clearly, a computer-administered and scored measure of health literacy would make is assessment more accessible in both clinical and research settings by reducing demands on clinician or researcher time while better standardizing the measure's administration. Integration of such a measure into an electronic health record might allow for inclusion of health literacy scores into patients' health records. This would transmit information about patients' level of health literacy directly to treating clinicians, allowing them to better understand patients' information needs. The automated assessment of health literacy might also allow for the automated tailoring of disease-related information, a strategy previously shown to be effective in influencing patient behavior,[20;21] and which may be effective in reducing health disparities.[22]

Pleasant et al.[23] argue that new measures of health literacy should be multidimensional and assess health literacy as a latent construct. A multidimensional approach would recognize that functional health literacy comprises a number of distinct skills or abilities, such as reading, listening, and performing quantitative operations.[1] Evaluation of latent constructs is frequently used in psychological assessment to study an ability or trait that cannot be directly measured. Multiple test items believed to be related are administered and then what they have in common is statistically extracted, usually with factor analysis. Many item response theory (IRT) models approach the measurement of abilities as latent constructs and have been used to develop assessments of health literacy.[24-26] Pleasant et al.[23] also suggest that assessments should recognize that measures are most likely to be accurate when they are similar to the context in which the actual behavior occurs. Assessment using a video simulation of a clinical encounter, for example, may be more accurate than asking for responses to written questions.

Jordan et al.16 report a review of existing health literacy measures and find many of them lacking in important measurement characteristics. These authors note the great variability in the content assessed by measures and the lack of a coherent conceptual model underlying them. Although measures such as the TOFHLA and the REALM provide descriptive score categories such as "adequate" or "inadequate" to assist in interpretation, the rationale for them is not clear. Jordan et al. also report limitations in the construct validity of measures, noting that the correlations of the measures with other measures of health literacy and reading are quite variable. These findings imply that different measures may actually evaluate different abilities and skills, calling into question their typical interpretation of measures of the same construct, an issue also raised by Haun et al.27 Finally, Jordan et al. assess the feasibility of actually using the measures they review, noting that the need for time, individual administration, and scoring is a substantial limitation that may limit their use.

Several researchers have addressed these limitations in developing new assessments of health literacy. Hahn et al.24;26 created a health literacy assessment using a touch screen computer format they call the "Health Literacy Assessment Using Talking Touchscreen Technology," or Health LiTT. Their measure, developed in Spanish and English26 allows for automated administration and scoring and was developed using IRT methods. Data on this measure's development in Spanish is limited, however, and the sample of Spanish-speaking adults used in development efforts was not clearly characterized as to bilingualism or linguistic preference. How the Spanish-speaking participants were chosen to be tested in Spanish or English is not clearly described, nor is their level of acculturation. The measure is not equivalent in Spanish and English as test stimuli differ in the two versions of the measure, limiting its usefulness in research, and both Spanish and English-speaking groups were patients in primary care with low levels of educational attainment. Although clearly a relevant population, the development of the measure with persons likely to have a limited range of ability may indicate that the measure will not function well in assessment of persons with higher levels of ability. The importance of understanding patients' English competence when information is delivered to non-native speakers has been shown in studies by several investigators.[28;29] The measure may thus replicate the commonly-observed ceiling effect from the TOFHLA. The Health LiTT measure is not based on a coherent theory or conceptual model of health literacy, although the authors link its development to an existing descriptive definition of health literacy[26]. Further, the reading comprehension section of this measure continues to rely on the cloze procedure which, as noted above, may result in items that are differentially more difficult for older participants. Finally, in a 2011 publication the authors report that the Health LiTT will be available through The Assessment Center (http://www.assessmentcenter.net), a free online resource that allows investigators to access a standardized set of measures for use in research. At the time of this writing, however, it is not available on this site. The actual availability of this measure for use is not clear.

Lee et al.[25] developed an instrument based on the REALM, selecting items based on analyses of DIF between Spanish- and English-speaking patients seen in a primary care clinic. As with other measures of health literacy, this measure continues to tap a narrow range of content and has limited demonstrations of its relation to other measures that might help establish its validity. It does not assess numeracy at all, and only provides a limited assessment of comprehension. It thus suffers from the other of the limitations others have criticized, including sampling a limited range of content, uncertain relation to actual health behaviors, and development on a small population of clinic patients.

A group at the Research Triangle Institute led by Lauren McCormack has also developed a new measure of health literacy, the Health Literacy Skills Instrument (HLSI).[30;31] This measure was developed using a rigorous psychometric approach and can be computer administered and scored. The development population was broader than that used to create most other measures (research volunteers vs. clinic patients in many other studies), and the development population was large (several thousand). Analyses of its validity have been presented.[30;32] The manual for this measure, however, does not provide directions for administering the measure either in person or by computer, raising questions about whether the measure would be reliable without a standard approach to administration.[31] The authors suggest that the measure can be administered as a paper and pencil test, but it uses an audio recording to assess listening comprehension and the requires access to several web pages to answer two questions, thus raising questions about how this might be possible. Such an administration would again not be standardized, raising questions about the validity of this form.

Although the article describing the measure states that five subscales can be constructed from the 25 items in the final measure, the final test manual provided by the authors does not describe how to score them nor do either of the articles describing its development and use provide data on the psychometric characteristics (reliability, validity) of the subscales. The measure's manual states that it assesses oral health literacy, and this statement appears to refer to a two items on the measure that require that the person assessed listen to a telephone menu recording and determine which button on the telephone to press. It thus assesses listening comprehension with two items. Similarly, the measure states that it assesses "information seeking skills" on the Internet, but this statement refers to two items in which a hyperlink is provided that takes the person assessed directly to a web page.[31] The two pages include calculators for calories burned during exercise and risk for heart attack. While these are useful information skills, these items do not actually assess an individual's ability to locate information on the Internet, an increasingly important skill.[33;34] Finally, the HLSI is not available in Spanish so that it may have limited usefulness with the most rapidly growing minority population in the United States.

This measure thus addresses many of the issues previously raised in critical evaluations of measures of health literacy. Its psychometric characteristics have been established, and it taps a wider range of content than other measures. It includes two items tapping listening comprehension, although it appears likely that these items cannot be used as a separate scale. The measure can be computer administered and scored, but no standard format for this administration is provided raising questions about the reliability of test scores that might result from diverse approaches to administration. It can be administered by computer, but as described it appears likely that this administration format requires the use of a computer mouse to answer questions and to navigate hyperlinks. Given the difficulty many elders and others with little computer experience have in using a computer mouse (and especially the fine psychomotor skills required to click the small dots used by this instrument to a preferred answer), it is likely that the format of administration as developed may place the very groups in which health literacy is most important at a disadvantage when responding to its questions. Although it includes items that mimic health-related calculators that might be found on the Internet, they do not actually assess Internet information search. As the web pages are on an external server, the ability to administer them requires and Internet connection and limits the ability of users to administer the measure by paper and pencil. Finally, the measure is brief, does not have separate subscales for skills such as reading, numeracy, and listening, and is not available in Spanish.

As summarized by Pleasant and McKinney15 and suggested by Jordan et al.16 many workers in the field have argued that new measures of health literacy should be developed that broaden the range of content assessed, are based on diverse groups, and have better-demonstrated psychometric characteristics. We are currently engaged in the development of a new measure of health literacy that addresses these criticisms. It samples a wide range of content chosen from the domains listed in the 2004 IOM report1 on the competencies needed for adequate health literacy. It is based on a coherent conceptual model of health literacy that has been developed based on our own and others' research. It includes items that assess prose, document, and quantitative literacies in each of the domains. It has been developed through a rigorous two-stage process in which items have been pilot tested, assessed for equivalence in both Spanish and English as well as in younger and older individuals, and has been subjected to assessments of construct and concurrent validity. It assesses not only reading and quantitative skills but also uses video simulations of healthcare related encounters to assess listening comprehension and to provide test stimuli that bear a close relation to the actual situations in which health literacy skills might be applied. By asking questions that assess expressive writing skills (by asking, for example, where certain kinds of information would be placed in a form) the measure indirectly assesses expressive written language skills. The purpose of this paper is to describe the initial development and testing of this new measure and provide preliminary data on its validity and reliability. The new measure utilizes a broad range of item formats and contents, includes listening comprehension, and has been developed in Spanish and English. The English project has been named Fostering Literacy for Good Health Today (FLIGHT) and the related Spanish project has been named Vive Desarollando Amplia Salud (VIDAS).

Methods

Overview

This section provides an overview of study procedures (see Figure). Test items were developed to sample a broad range of health-related content in Spanish and English. The sample on which the measure is validated is purposefully drawn from a range of abilities and backgrounds as evidenced by participants' occupations and educations. In order to accurately characterize Spanish-speaking participants, we developed a procedure to assess language dominance in Spanish-English bilinguals. Items in both languages were created to minimize the impact of regional usage and data analyses employ a combination of classical test theory35-37 and item response theory19 techniques.

In Phase 1, a pool of candidate items was administered to Spanish and English speakers, with approximately one-half of each group aged 50 years or older. Items were screened for difficulty and discrimination (correlation with total score) and for age- and language-associated DIF. The original pool of items was reduced and some new items were written to enhance the total scale's range of content and difficulty. In Phase 2 (currently in progress with initial results presented here), items developed in Phase 1 are administered to an age-stratified sample of community-dwelling Spanish and English speakers along with measures chosen to establish the new scale's validity. This paper presents information on the first 93 Spanish- and 105 English-speaking participants who have completed Phase 2.

Computer Delivered Format

In order to ensure that the resulting measure will be inexpensive and easily deployed, it has been developed using off-the-shelf touch-screen computers that are readily available and reasonably priced (HP TouchSmart®; Hewlett-Packard Corporation, Palo Alto, CA). These computers have large touch screens running the Windows® operating system (20 inch diagonal measurement) and include self-contained speakers that allow participants to hear all items as they are presented. In another project, we had done extensive user testing with the general format of touch screen interface, iteratively testing the interface, modifying it in response to user comments, and then retesting it.38;39 In Phase 1, we used the previously developed touchscreen format. Interviews after each participant completed the phase 1 focused on possible usability and navigation issues as well as on the format and content of the questions.

Item Development

A framework for item development was created based on the domains of literacy skills needed for health as outlined in the 2004 Institute of Medicine (IOM) report.1 For each of the seven health-related goals listed in the Report (left column in Table 1) items were created in one of the three formats commonly used in assessing literacy--prose, document, and quantitative.40 A 7 X 3 item content matrix was created and used as a guide in item development (Table 1). Candidate items were developed by individ-
ual

Insert Table 1 about here

---

team members and reviewed by the entire team. Members represent a range of health professions including medicine, nursing, social work, pharmacy, and psychology. Each team member has extensive experience in clinical work and thus is familiar with the types of clinical problems encountered by patients in obtaining health care. The lead investigator (RO) has extensive experience with psychometric scale development with multiple publications on the subject. The team includes a psychologist with a strong background in multicultural and multilingual assessment (AA) who also has published multiple articles on psychometric assessment. Other members of the team have had extensive experience in patient education and assessment.

Some items were first created in Spanish and then translated into English, while others were created in English and translated. A guiding principle in item development was to create items that would be culturally and linguistically equivalent rather than word-for-word translations.41 From the project's inception, word and item selection have focused on use of high-frequency words and terms to ensure that participants would understand all questions. Care was taken to use words in both languages that would be understood by persons of varying socioeconomic and educational levels and that were not region- or nation-specific.

Items developed within the 7 x 3 content matrix targeted the component skills of literacy (conceptual knowledge, listening and speaking, writing, reading, and numeracy) as outlined in the IOM report.1 For example, to assess conceptual knowledge, items that tapped basic health facts were created (e.g., "Hemoglobin A1C measures which of the following?"). Listening comprehension was assessed using 60-90 second videos of simulated interactions with health care providers or presentations of health information. For example, one video showed an encounter in which a patient was given a new medication and directions for its use, and another simulated a TV news presentation on finding health information on the Internet. After viewing, participants responded to multiple choice questions. It was not possible to directly assess participants' oral expression, but questions were created that presented problems that could only be solved by communicating with providers (e.g., "Arthur doesn't understand what the doctor says. What can he do?").

Written expression was assessed as document literacy through questions evaluating participants' ability to complete materials such as insurance forms. Navigating the health care system included interpreting hospital maps; some documents and maps included items that asked participants to respond by tapping on the appropriate area of the screen (e.g., "Tap on the area where you would find information on how to use toothpaste with a 4 year old"). Reading comprehension was assessed through questions about passages of varying difficulty levels, and numeracy was assessed through items demanding reading, arithmetic computation and decision making based on probabilities. Approximately ten items were created for each element in the item content matrix resulting in 208 candidate items.

Phase 1: Initial Item Testing

This base group of items was administered to 69 Spanish- and 73 English-speaking participants. Language dominance of Spanish-speaking participants who indicated that they also spoke English was assessed by comparing their performance on the relative proficiency indices (RPI) of the reading and listening comprehension subtests of the Woodcock-Johnson (English) and the Woodcock-Muñoz (Spanish) Psycho-Educational Batteries (Rolling Meadows, IL: Riverside Publishing). Level of acculturation was assessed using the Marin Acculturation Scale.42 Most participants showed clear superiority in one language or the other (i.e., more than one standard deviation difference in RPI scores), including those who indicated they had proficiency in both languages. Only those participants who showed clear evidence of greater proficiency in Spanish completed the Spanish assessment. The importance of actually assessing Hispanic participants' language skills is underscored by a study that showed that Hispanics who state they are fluent in English may function at lower levels compared to native English speakers.29

Almost half of each language group was 50 years of age or older (30 of 69 Spanish and 29 of 73 English speakers) allowing for the assessment of language- and age-related DIF. As discussed above, we believed that this issue was important in light of our finding that almost one-half of the items on the reading comprehension scale of the TOFHLA showed evidence of age-related DIF. After responding to all items, participants completed interviews during which items were reviewed with them for problems in clarity and to assess whether the items actually measured what was intended. Initial analyses were completed using jMetrik (www.itemanalysis.com), assessing item difficulties, discriminations (item-total correlations), and the presence of DIF. The Mantel-Haenszel chi-square statistic as well as the Educational Testing Service grading system43 were used to evaluate DIF, supplemented by review of nonparametric item response curves.

In creating the final item pool for further study, some items were eliminated due language-related DIF, while other items were rewritten after team consultation. No items showed substantial age-related DIF, supporting our decision to avoid using the cloze response procedure used in other measures, as it may bias items against older individuals. A number of items were either low or mid-range in difficulty; many of these were eliminated when their content or format duplicated other items. Data from interviews were used to rewrite items when participants indicated that an item was confusing or when the interviews showed that the item did not actually assess its target skill. Several new items were created in this phase in order to broaden the range of content covered and provide items with greater difficulties. Although these items were not subjected to the same developmental testing as other from Phase 1, these will be assessed for psychometric characteristics prior to inclusion in a final measure. This procedure resulted in the 98 items being used in Phase 2.

Phase 2: Further Development and Testing

The purpose of this phase is to validate the new health literacy measure by assessing its relations to other measures of health literacy and of participants' health. A purposive sample with a range of abilities (based on education and occupation) is being recruited over specific age ranges. This strategy is likely to be the most efficient approach to obtain optimal item statistics with relatively small samples.[44;45] Interested participants are first screened for cognitive status using the Short Portable Mental Status Questionnaire[46] and paragraphs from the Wechsler Memory Scale[47] using cut off scores previously developed in a study of computer use in elderly participants (S. Czaja, unpublished data). Participants are also screened for vision and auditory abilities using a visual screener and auditory comprehension of material presented over headphones calibrated using a handheld decibel meter (Extech Model 407730, Extech Instruments, Waltham MA). Spanish-speaking participants are being recruited from a several different national backgrounds including the countries of Central and South America as well as the US and Mexico. The language of assessment is determined using the procedure developed in Phase 1, using the language preference subscale of the Marin Acculturation Scale[42] supplemented with additional testing when participants indicate significant use of both languages.

In addition to the new health literacy items, participants complete a battery of existing health literacy measures (TOFHLA in both Spanish and English; REALM or SAHLSA, and the self-report questions developed by Chew et al.[48]), literacy- and numeracy-related academic skills and basic cognitive abilities. They also provide information on health status, health-related quality of life, and health service utilization. Participants complete assessments in two sessions (individually-administered cognitive and health literacy measures in one, questionnaires and the health literacy measures administered by touch screen computer in the other) with order of administration of each session randomly counterbalanced to account for order effects. Because of the length of assessment sessions, participants can complete both either in a single day (during which they take at least a one-hour break for lunch) or on two days. Measures have been selected to allow the evaluation of the relation of the new measure to existing assessments of health literacy, basic cognitive skills, relevant academic skills such as reading and math skills, and health status variables. The REALM assesses health literacy based on an individuals' ability to read orthographically-irregular words in English. As Spanish has few orthographically-irregular words, the SAHLSA is administered to Spanish speakers as the closest equivalent. Participants also respond to the self-report health literacy screening questions developed by Chew et al.[48] and evaluated in English and Spanish by Sarkar et al.[49]

Sample

Participants are recruited via flyers, presentations at community organizations, and by recruitment from previous studies. Sampling focuses on recruiting groups of Spanish- and English-speaking participants in the age ranges 18-30; 31-40; 41-50; 51-60; 61-70; 71-80; and 81 years and older. Recruitment is targeted to various socioeconomic, occupational, and educational backgrounds (e.g., ranging from grade school to doctoral-level graduate education) and, in the case of Spanish-speaking participants, to a range of national origins (Central and South America as well as Spain, Mexico and the US). Participants are compensated $80.00 for each session completed. Participants who complete the study in a single day are provided with lunch, and funds are available to reimburse participants for their use of public transportation. All participants have completed both sessions and none has dropped out of the study between sessions.

Data Analyses

Initial analyses assessed each item's relation to overall ability (item discrimination, evaluated as an item-total correlation greater than 0.20) and the extent to which each was equivalent in Spanish and English. Inspection of nonparametric item response curves, chi square testing for DIF, and ETS classification, in which items are rated depending on the degree and clinical significance of the DIF[40] were performed. Further analyses included exploratory and confirmatory factor analyses using MPlus (Los

Angeles: Muthén and Muthén) and focused on choosing items that were clearly related to content-defined scales (i.e., an item that required an arithmetic computation was related to the numeracy scale). These analyses first established that the instrument was multifactorial (via assessment of the results of exploratory factor analyses based on fit indices and the scree plot of eigenvalues for exploratory models and with multiple factors and fit indices in confirmatory models). Confirmatory models then evaluated a multifactor model with separate scales reflecting general health literacy (HL), numeracy (NUM), listening comprehension (LIS), and conceptual knowledge of health-related facts (FACT). The equivalence of the factor model for both Spanish and English speakers was assessed in separate confirmatory factor analyses for each language group as well as in the combined sample.

Development of Scales

Scales of the measure were developed through a combined process of exploratory and confirmatory factor analysis and rational scale construction. Factor models were evaluated in both language groups separately and items that did not load significantly on any factor were eliminated. Four scales were developed to reflect general health literacy, numeracy, listening comprehension based on responses to video-related items, and conceptual knowledge based on responses to questions that require only knowledge of specific health-related facts (e.g., "Hemoglobin A1C measures which of the following?"). The fit of this four-factor model was evaluated separately for both Spanish- and English-speaking participants as well as in the combined sample.

Reliability and Validity

Cronbach's alpha and correlations of the new measure's scales with the TOFHLA, REALM, SAHLSA, and self-report questions were calculated in order to evaluate the new measure's reliability and concurrent validity. Known groups validity was assessed by assigning participants to groups based on their total TOFHLA score and evaluating the ability of the general health literacy scale (HL) to differentiate among them.

Participant Satisfaction

After completing the new measure, participants completed a questionnaire based on the Technology Acceptance Model[50] that asked for their ratings of the measure's usefulness, ease of use, enjoyment, and whether they would use it again.

All study procedures were completed under a protocol approved by the Institutional Review Board of Nova Southeastern University.

RESULTS

Phase 1

Demographic data for phase 1 are presented in the top portion of Table 2. In Phase 1, only data on participant age, race, ethnicity, and education were collected as the primary purpose of this phase to screen a larger number of items in order to have a substantial number for use in the validation study in Phase 2. The 208 items administered in this phase were evaluated to assess their difficulties, discriminations, and both age- and language-related DIF. Of the 208 items, 113 items were deleted due to low discriminations (i.e., low relation to overall health literacy), presence of language-related DIF, or a combination of low difficulty and redundant content. When several items tapped similar content or skill and had similar levels of difficulty, items were chosen according to the more nearly unique content or for greater difficulty.

Phase 2

Demographic data for the samples (93 Spanish- and 105 English-speaking participants) are presented in Table 2. All Spanish-speaking participants described their racial background as white, consistent with findings from the US Census[51] while English-speaking participants were African American, Afro Caribbean, white, and Asian. Consistent with our sampling strategy, the average age of our participants is approximately 50, and the average level of education was equivalent to having completed high school. Our actual recruitment by target age groups is also included in this table.

Insert Table 2 about here

Scale Development

Initial exploratory factor analyses suggested the presence of more than one factor underlying our data. Scales (HL, NUM, LIS, or FACT) were created based on results of the preliminary factor analysis and item content and format while eliminating items with low relations (item loadings) to any of the scales. Confirmatory analyses indicated that some items from the NUM, LIS, and FACT scales also were related to general health literacy and were included in HL as well as the other scales. The fit of the resulting factor models was assessed in confirmatory analyses that evaluated progressively more complex models (encompassing first HL, then adding NUM, then FACT, and then LIS). Fit for the final four-factor model in the combined sample was good, with a nonsignificant chi-square value ($\chi2$ [df =2,676] = 2759.22, $p = 0.13$), an RMSEA value of 0.01, and a confirmatory fit index value of 0.97.

Factor scores for each factor in the combined group were calculated and used in analyses of correlations between the new measure's scales and other measures of health literacy. After scale development, MIMIC52 models evaluated whether any items continued to show language-related DIF; no remaining items showed significant DIF. The final scales are listed in Table 3 along with example item objectives and measures

---

Insert Table 3 about here

---

of scale reliability for each language group as well as for the entire sample. The HL and NUM scales have acceptable reliabilities, but the FACT and LIS scale have borderline to low reliabilities. This suggests that further work is needed in developing these scales, although we note that some items from each scale contribute to the HL scale which has an acceptable reliability. We suggest regarding these scales as experimental pending further development.

Scale intercorrelations and correlations with other measures of health literacy are presented in Table 4. The new measures' scales are significantly intercorrelated reflecting the common composition of HL with the other scales (some items were common to HL and the other scales) while correlations among other scales (NUM, FACT, and LIS) are not influenced by common items (i.e., no items loaded on pairs of

---

Insert Table 4 about here

---

these factors). Thirteen items from the FACT scale and 11 items from LIS are included in the HL subscale. This strategy was employed in order to allow us to develop a broad general health literacy scale based on the items that were most closely related to overall health literacy as suggested by factor analyses.

The new measure's scales are also related to other measures of health literacy. HL correlated significantly ($p < 0.01$) with the TOFHLA reading and numeracy scales, the REALM, the SAHLSA, and the self-report items. Each of the remaining scales was correlated significantly with the TOFHLA, REALM, and SAHLSA. The FACT and LIS scales are significantly correlated with other measures (TOFHLA, REALM, and the SAHLSA) suggesting that the constructs they measure (health-related knowledge and listening comprehension) are related to health literacy in spite of the scales' low reliabilities. The correlations of the new measure's scales with existing measures of health literacy are similar to the correlations found between existing measures, suggesting that the new measure has substantial concurrent validity.

Known Groups Validity

In order to further assess the usefulness of the HL scale, we evaluated its ability to differentiate among participants assigned to groups based on their scores on the TOFHLA. We grouped participants in three groups: those with total TOFHLA scores less than 91 (of 100), those with total scores between 91 and 95, and those with scores greater than 95. Analysis of variance (ANOVA) models were assessed separately for English and Spanish participants.

Of the English speaking participants, 19 were in the group with scores less than 91, 29 were in the group with scores between 91 and 95, and 53 were in the group with scores greater than 95. The ANOVA model for English speakers showed that the HL scale scores differed significantly across groups ($F [2,101] = 23.74$, $p < 0.001$). Post-hoc analyses showed that all groups differed significantly from each other (all $ps < 0.01$).

For Spanish speaking participants, 53 participants were in the group with scores less than 91, 22 were in the group with scores from 91 to 95, and 17 were in the group with scores greater than 95. The model for this group also showed that the HL scale scores differed significantly across groups ($F [2,92] = 24.72$, $p < 0.001$). Post-hoc analyses again showed that all groups differed significantly from each other (all $ps < 0.01$).

Participant Satisfaction

Participants' average ratings of the measure's usefulness on a scale from 0 to 6 was 5.03 (SD = 1.25). Their mean rating of how easy it was to use was 5.37 (SD = 0.95). Participants' ratings of enjoyment in using the measure were also positive (5.00, SD = 1.03) as were their ratings on items asking if they would use the measure again (5.08, SD = 0.73). Participants' ratings of usefulness, ease of use, enjoyment, or intent to use in the future were not related to the language in which they completed the measure (t-tests comparing language groups; all ps > 0.10).

Discussion

The purpose of this study has been to develop and validate a computer-administered measure of health literacy. In this study, health literacy is defined more broadly than in other measures to encompass the domains of content and skills outlined in the 2004 IOM report 1 while reflecting the literacy formats of other measures 40;53. Our approach has focused on creating a measure that assesses as broad a range of health literacy skills as possible within the constraints of computer-administration and scoring. It is thus able to evaluate participants' comprehension of written language, understanding of health-related documents, and ability to use quantitative skills in performing health-related tasks and making probability-based judgments. By including video vignettes of health-related situations such as an encounter with a provider giving instructions for a new medication, it also assesses listening comprehension. The new HL scale includes items related to finding health information on the Internet making it one of the first measures to evaluate these skills. Through the development process described in this paper, it has been possible to create a multidimensional assessment instrument that has significant relations to other measures, suggesting that it has concurrent validity. Participants' reactions to using the measure have been uniformly positive, showing that it may be acceptable for more general use.

Our central purpose in developing FLIGHT/VIDAS has been to develop a measure of health literacy that would address the criticisms of existing measures, as summarized in several reviews.[16;23] Core issues identified by researchers have been the range of content assessed by measures, their psychometric characteristics such as reliability and validity, relation to actual health behaviors, lack of measures that are equivalent in both Spanish and English, and lack of basis in an actual theory or model of health literacy with the apparent result that different measures of "health literacy" may actually assess different things.[27] In the FLIGHT/VIDAS project, we have addressed each of these issues by developing and evaluating a model of health literacy, by employing rigorous methods and testing in item and scale development while creating items with a broad range of content and response formats, including video simulations of actual health encounters, developing the measure simultaneously in both Spanish and English, and including a range of measures for use in validating the new measure.

Some time ago, Baker[14] noted that it would be helpful to have a measure of conceptual knowledge of health and illness. In this project, we have attempted to develop just such a measure in the FACT scale that assesses health-related conceptual knowledge. Analyses suggest that this initial attempt has been partially successful. The FACT scale's reliability is lower than may be desirable, but it is significantly correlated with other measures of health literacy. Because of its clear content validity, it may be useful for research in which the role of cognitive skills and disease-related knowledge in health literacy are examined. Chin et al.[54] for example, used this strategy. Understanding the relation of specific disease knowledge to health literacy may facilitate the development of measures in which general skills such as reading or numeracy are integrated with disease-related knowledge. Researchers have successfully employed this strategy in developing disease-specific health literacy measures[55] and it may also be useful in guiding the development of interventions.

The model of health literacy underlying FLIGHT/VIDAS explicitly includes conceptual knowledge as an aspect of health literacy. While it may be possible to separate conceptual knowledge from other health literacy skills, our decision to include health-related conceptual knowledge is grounded in research showing that basic knowledge interacts with reading or listening skills in producing competent performances, whether in basic reading among school children[56;57] or in complex activities such as sight reading piano music,[58] and playing chess.[59] Other research has supported this view in studying health literacy.[54] Implicit in this view of health literacy is that it reflects the ability to carry out complex activities that may include using existing information and skills to solve new problems.[60] Assessing core conceptual knowledge related to healthcare, from this point of view, is essential to understanding the ways in which health literacy affects the ability to obtain and use health information.

This development process is similar to that taken by others in creating new measures of health literacy. Using IRT techniques and sampling Spanish and English speakers, Hahn and colleagues[24;26] and Lee and colleagues[25] have developed measures of health literacy that can be used in both languages and which have clearly defined psychometric properties. Differences in our approach compared to the measure described by Hahn et al., Health LiTT, include the response formats used (our measure does not use the cloze procedure as it may have a differential impact on older persons), our focus on equivalence of items in both languages (Health LiTT prose passages are different and nonequivalent in the Spanish and English versions), and the use of a sample drawn from the community rather than from clinics. For the new scale we developed a method to assess participants' language dominance (the language in which they clearly performed better) and assessed participants in that language so that those who completed the Spanish language version of the measure are clearly characterized as to linguistic competence and level of acculturation. As reported by Aguirre et al.[28] and Downey and Zun[29] Hispanics who complete assessments in English may be at a disadvantage to non-Hispanics whose native language is English, even when they appear to be able to speak and understand English. As there are wide variations in the cultural and linguistic backgrounds of individuals from Spanish-speaking countries who live in the US,[61] the assessment of the Spanish-language items with individuals from a number of different Spanish-speaking countries may be an important aspect of making the measure more generally useful.

While the Health LiTT may be more useful in assessing whether patients have deficiencies in health literacy (for example, the authors indicate that they focused mainly on items in the range of 6th to 11th grade equivalent difficulties; see Yost et al.,[26] p. 297), our measure may be more relevant to understanding health literacy in the general population, especially in normal elderly (because the new measure does not use the cloze procedure) and younger and healthier individuals (because they have been included in our development and validation samples).

The instrument developed by Lee et al.[25] may be useful for persons interested in assessing patients' health literacy as their ability to recognize health-related words and link those words to their meanings. This measure is brief and may be used for screening, but it assesses a smaller range of health literacy skills (notably, it does not include numeracy) and is not computer administered or scored. Each of these measures, including the one reported upon here, have strengths and weaknesses. We suggest that advantages of the new measure are that it assesses a broad range of skills, does not use the cloze procedure, and includes items that are equivalent in both Spanish and English.

Limitations of our approach include the indirect assessment of oral expression in the measure (only measured by asking participants to imagine their responses to problematic encounters with providers and not constituting a separate scale), the current modest sample size, and the need to administer the measure by way of computers. While computers are available in many clinical and research settings, they may not be available in many other settings in which health literacy might be assessed. It may be useful to develop a measure that can be administered on more convenient portable devices such as the iPad®, and our long-term development plans include developing such a version. Another important limitation of the FACT and LIS scales are their low reliabilities in one or both language groups. Because of their clear content validity and relation to other measures of health literacy, these scales may be useful for research purposes. They should be regarded as experimental and potentially useful pending further development.

The purpose of this study is thus to develop and validate an innovative computer-administered measure of health literacy that assesses a broad range of health literacy skills within the constraints of a computer-administered measure. It is anticipated that by expanding the range of skills assessed, the new measure may have wider usefulness and better ability to predict important health-related outcomes. Two new scales in this measure, those assessing health-related conceptual knowledge (FACT) and listening comprehension (LIS), may provide information useful in developing a broader understanding of which skills are most important in particular contexts. For example, listening comprehension might be important in patients' ability to benefit from typical health encounters that rely heavily on clinicians' oral communication of information, while written and numeracy skills might be related to patients' success at following written treatment guidelines or becoming involved in health promotion activities. The new measure's inclusion of items related to health information on the Internet may also be a useful addition to health literacy assessment that merits further exploration as technology becomes more and more important in health care. Given the new measures' relation to existing measures, we believe that we have created a useful and valid measure of health literacy skills. Data collection in phase 2 is continuing and will be completed in 2014. We anticipate being able to make the measure available shortly thereafter.

DISCLOSURES

All authors state that they have no conflicts of interest to disclose.

ACKNOWLEDGEMENT

The study described in this paper was supported by grant R01HL096578 to Dr. Ownby from the National Heart, Lung, and Blood Institute.

Reference List

(1) Nielsen-Bohlman L, Panzer AM, Kindig DA. Health literacy: A prescription to end confusion. 2004. Washington DC, National Academies Press.

Ref Type: Edited Book

(2) Berkman ND, Sheridan SL, Donahue KE, Halpern DJ, Crotty K. Low health literacy and health outcomes: an updated systematic review. Ann Intern Med 2011;155:97-107.

(3) Dewalt DA, Berkman ND, Sheridan S, Lohr KN, Pignone MP. Literacy and health outcomes: a systematic review of the literature. J Gen Intern Med 2004;19:1228-1239.

(4) Bostock S, Steptoe A. Association between low functional health literacy and mortality in older adults: longitudinal cohort study. BMJ 2012;344:e1602.

(5) Sudore RL, Yaffe K, Satterfield S et al. Limited literacy and mortality in the elderly: the health, aging, and body composition study. J Gen Intern Med 2006;21:806-812.

(6) Ownby RL, Waldrop-Valverde D, Jacobs RJ, Caballero J. Baseline medication adherence and response to an electronically-delivered health literacy intervention targeting adherence. Neurobehavioral HIV Medicine 2012;4:113-121.

(7) Sheridan SL, Halpern DJ, Viera AJ, Berkman ND, Donahue KE, Crotty K. Interventions for individuals with low health literacy: a sys-

tematic review. J Health Commun 2011;16 Suppl 3:30-54.

(8) Osborn CY, Cavanaugh K, Wallston KA et al. Health literacy explains racial disparities in diabetes medication adherence. J Health Commun 2011;16 Suppl 3:268-278.

(9) Waldrop-Valverde D, Osborn CY, Rodriguez A, Rothman RL, Kumar M, Jones DL. Numeracy skills explain racial differences in HIV medication management. AIDS Behav 2010;14:799-806.

(10) Parker RM, Baker DW, Williams MV, Nurss JR. The Test of Functional Health Literacy in Adults: A new instrument for measuring patients' literacy skills. J Gen Intern Med 1995;10:537-541.

(11) Murphy PW, Davis TC, Long SW, Jackson RH, Decker BC. Rapid Estimate of Adult Literacy in Medicine (REALM): A quick reading test for patients. Journal of Reading 1993;37:124-130.

(12) Weiss BD, Mays MZ, Martz W et al. Quick assessment of literacy in primary care: the newest vital sign. Ann Fam Med 2005;3:514-522.

(13) Baker DW, Williams MV, Parker RM, Gazmararian JA, Nurss J. Development of a brief test to measure functional health literacy. Patient Educ Couns 1999;38:33-42.

(14) Baker DW. The meaning and the measure of health literacy. J Gen Intern Med 2006;21:878-883.

(15) Pleasant A, McKinney J. Coming to consensus on health literacy measurement: an online discussion and consensus-gauging process. Nurs Outlook 2011;59:95-106.

(16) Jordan JE, Osborne RH, Buchbinder R. Critical appraisal of health literacy indices revealed variable underlying constructs, narrow content and psychometric weaknesses. J Clin Epidemiol 2011;64:366-379.

(17) Ackerman PL, Beier ME, Bowen KR. Explorations of crys-

tallized intelligence: Completion tests, cloze tests, and knowledge. Learning and Individual Differences 2000;12:105-121.

(18) Ackerman PL, Cianciolo AT. Cognitive, perceptual-speed, and psychomotor determinants of individual differences during skill acquisition. J Exp Psychol Appl 2000;6:259-290.

(19) Embretson SE, Reise SP. Item response theory for psychologists. Mahwah, NJ: Lawrence Erlbaum, 2000.

(20) Noar SM, Benac CN, Harris MS. Does tailoring matter? Meta-analytic review of tailored print health behavior change interventions. Psychol Bull 2007;133:673-693.

(21) Ownby RL, Hertzog C, Czaja SJ. Tailored information and automated reminding to improve medication adherence in Spanish- and English-speaking elders treater for memory impairment. Clinical Gerontologist 2012;35:221-238.

(22) Jerant A, Sohler N, Fiscella K, Franks B, Franks P. Tailored interactive multimedia computer programs to reduce health disparities: opportunities and challenges. Patient Educ Couns 2011;85:323-330.

(23) Pleasant A, McKinney J, Rikard RV. Health literacy measurement: a proposed research agenda. J Health Commun 2011;16 Suppl 3:11-21.

(24) Hahn EA, Choi SW, Griffith JW, Yost KJ, Baker DW. Health literacy assessment using talking touchscreen technology (Health LiTT): a new item response theory-based measure of health literacy. J Health Commun 2011;16 Suppl 3:150-162.

(25) Lee SY, Stucky BD, Lee JY, Rozier RG, Bender DE. Short Assessment of Health Literacy-Spanish and English: a comparable test of health literacy for Spanish and English speakers. Health Serv Res 2010;45:1105-1120.

(26) Yost KJ, Webster K, Baker DW, Choi SW, Bode RK, Hahn EA. Bilingual health literacy assessment using the Talking Touchscreen/la Pantalla Parlanchina: Development and pilot testing. Patient Educ Couns 2009;75:295-301.

(27) Haun J, Luther S, Dodd V, Donaldson P. Measurement variation across health literacy assessments: implications for assessment selection in research and practice. J Health Commun 2012;17 Suppl 3:141-159.

(28) Aguirre AC, Ebrahim N, Shea JA. Performance of the English and Spanish S-TOFHLA among publicly insured Medicaid and Medicare patients. Patient Educ Couns 2005;56:332-339.

(29) Zun LS, Sadoun T, Downey L. English-language competency of self-declared English-speaking Hispanic patients using written tests of health literacy. J Natl Med Assoc 2006;98:912-917.

(30) McCormack L, Bann C, Squiers L et al. Measuring health literacy: a pilot study of a new skills-based instrument. J Health Commun 2010;15 Suppl 2:51-71.

(31) McCormack L. Health literacy skills instrument: User guide. Research Triangle Park, NC: RTI International. Available at http:// http://www.rti.org/page.cfm?objectid=66F893E4-5056-B100-0C834F234F368198. Accessed May 20, 2013.

(32) Bann CM, McCormack LA, Berkman ND, Squiers LB. The Health Literacy Skills Instrument: a 10-item short form. J Health Commun 2012;17 Suppl 3:191-202.

(33) Ownby RL. Technology and psychogeriatrics: Health and computer literacy. International Psychogeriatrics. In press.

(34) Ownby RL, Czaja SJ. Healthcare website design for the elderly: improving usability. AMIA Annu Symp Proc 2003;960.

(35) DeVellis RF. Classical test theory. Med Care 2006;44:S50-S59.

(36) Gulliksen H. Theory of mental tests. New York: Wiley, 1950.

(37) Lord FM, Novick MR. Statistical theories of mental test scores. Boston, MA: Addison-Wesley, 1968.

(38) Ownby RL, Waldrop-Valverde D, Jacobs RJ, Caballero J. Baseline medication adherence and response to an electronically-delivered health literacy intervention targeting adherence. Neurobehavioral HIV Medicine 2012;4:113-121.

(39) Ownby RL, Waldrop-Valverde D, Jacobs RJ, Acevedo A, Caballero J. Cost effectiveness of a computer-delivered intervention to improve HIV medication adherence. BMC Medical Informatics and Decision Making 2013;13:29.

(40) Kirsch I. The International Adult Literacy Survey (IALS): Understanding what was measured. Princeton, NJ: Educational Testing Service, 2001.

(41) Acevedo A, Krueger KR, Navarro E et al. The Spanish translation and adaptation of the Uniform Data Set of the National Institute on Aging Alzheimer's Disease Centers. Alzheimer Dis Assoc Disord 2009;23:102-109.

(42) Marin G, Sabogal F, Marin BV, Otero-Sabogal R, Perez-Stable EJ. Development of a short acculturation scale for Hispanics. Hispanic Journal of Behavioral Sciences 1987;9:183-205.

(43) Zwick R. A review of ETS differential item functioning assessment procedures: Flagging rules, minimum sample size requirements, and criterion refinement. Princeton, NJ: Educational Testing Service, 2012.

(44) Orlando M. Critical issues to address when applying item response theory (IRT) models. Paper presented at the conference Advanc-

es in Health Outcomes Measurement: Exploring the Current State and the Future of Item Response Theory, Item Banks, and Computer-Adaptive Testing, Bethesda, MD, June. 2004.

(45) Wingersky MS, Lord FM. An investigation of methods for reducing sampling error in certain IRT procedures. Applied Psychological Measurement 1984;8:347-364.

(46) Pfeiffer E. A short portable mental status questionnaire for the assessment of organic brain deficit in elderly patients. J Am Geriatr Soc 1975;23:433-441.

(47) Wechsler D. Manual for the Wechsler Memory Scale, Fourth edition. San Antonio, TX: Psychological Corporation/Pearson Assessment, 2008.

(48) Chew LD, Griffin JM, Partin MR et al. Validation of screening questions for limited health literacy in a large VA outpatient population. J Gen Intern Med 2008;23:561-566.

(49) Sarkar U, Schillinger D, Lopez A, Sudore R. Validation of self-reported health literacy questions among diverse English and Spanish-speaking populations. J Gen Intern Med 2011;26:265-271.

(50) Venkatesh V. Determinants of perceived ease of use: Integrating control, intrinsic motivation, and emotion into the Technology Acceptance Model. Information Systems Research 2000;11:342.

(51) Ennis SR, Rios-Vargas M, Albert NG. The Hispanic population: 2010. Washington, DC: US Department of Commerce, US Census Bureau, 2011.

(52) Fleishman JA. Using MIMIC models to assess the influence of differential item functioning. Paper presented at the conference Advances in Health Outcomes Measurement: Exploring the Current State and the Future of Item Response Theory, Item Banks, and Computer-Adaptive

Testing, Bethesda, MD, June. 2004.

(53) White S, Dillow S. Key concepts and features of the 2003 National Assessment of Adult Literacy (NCES 2006-471). Washington DC: US Department of Education, National Center for Educational Statistics, 2005.

(54) Chin J, Morrow DG, Stine-Morrow EA, Conner-Garcia T, Graumlich JF, Murray MD. The process-knowledge model of health literacy: evidence from a componential analysis of two commonly used measures. J Health Commun 2011;16 Suppl 3:222-241.

(55) Ownby RL, Waldrop-Valverde D, Hardigan P, Caballero J, Jacobs R, Acevedo A. Development and validation of a brief computer-administered HIV-related health literacy scale (HIV-HL). AIDS Behav 2013;17:710-718.

(56) Beck IL, Perfetti CA, McKeown MG. Effects of long-term vocabulary instruction on lexical access and reading comoprehension. Journal of Educational Psychology 1982;74:506-521.

(57) Nagy WE. Teaching vocabulary to improve reading comprehension. Urbana, IL: National Council of Teachers of English, 1988.

(58) Meinz EJ, Hambrick DZ. Deliberate practice is necessary but not sufficient to explain individual differences in piano sight-reading skill: the role of working memory capacity. Psychol Sci 2010;21:914-919.

(59) Hambrick DZ, Meinz EJ. Limits on the predictive power of domain-specific experience and knowledge in skilled performance. Curr Dir Psychol Sci 2011;20:275-279.

(60) Ownby RL, Waldrop-Valverde D. Health literacy is related to problem solving. Paper presented at the Health Literacy Research Conference. Washington DC: 2009.

(61) Motel S, Patten E. The 10 largest Hispanic origin groups: Characteristics, rankings, top counties. Washington, DC: Pew Research Center., 2012.

Table 1. Item content examples by IOM reports domains (Nielsen-Bohlman et al., 2004) and ETS formats (Kirsch, 2001)

Goals	Prose
Health promotion	Read a passage on exercise and identify desirable duration of exercise
Understand health information	Read a passage on risk factors for diabetes and identify relevant behaviors that would reduce someone's risk
Apply health information	After being provided with information on physical activity guidelines, identify appropriate exercise duration and frequencies
Navigate the health care system	After reading an informational brochure, be able to describe how specific health care services are covered by an insurance program
Participate in encounters with health care professionals	After viewing a video of a person's encounter with a physician providing a new medicine, identify information provided by the physician about dosage and schedule
Give informed consent	After reading information about a colonoscopy, describe the risks and benefits of the procedure
Understand rights	After reading an explanation of benefits, correctly identify the procedure to appeal a denial of benefits

Document	Quantitative
Make menu choices based on fat and sodium guidelines	Calculate the number of grams of fat in a package of a product given a per serving value
Given a checklist of risk factors for diabetes, be able to complete a checklist of risk factors for the disease	Given information on normal and abnormal blood glucose levels, identify normal and abnormal levels
Given narrative information on exercise frequency and intensity, complete an exercise log	Calculate the number of calories used during exercise give a table of exercises, times, and values; Use Internet based calculator to calculate body mass index
Review information from a table on dates and times for applying for specific health care benefits	Calculate relative costs of two insurance plans
After viewing a video describing how to apply for long term care insurance, fill out an application	After viewing a video that presents information on desirable weights, calculate one's own body mass index
After viewing a video that presents information on informed consent for a clinical study, describe its risks and benefits.	Given a graphical representation of the probability of a medication side effect, correctly identify how likely its occurrence will be.
Given an insurance explanation of benefits on an insurance payment statement, identify an inappropriate denial	After viewing a video presentation on patient rights, correctly determine the number of options available to access services

Table 2. Descriptive statistics for Phase 1 and 2 samples		
	Phase 1	
	Spanish	English
Gender M/F	22/50	64/50
Hispanic	72	12
African American		51
Afro Caribbean		12
Asian/Pacific Islander		
White	72	51
Continuous variables: Means (standard deviations)		
Age	47.0 (14.6)	47.5 (12.7)
Education	14.4 (2.6)	13.5 (2.0)
	Phase 2	
	Spanish	English
Gender M/F	41/52	52/53
Hispanic	93	3
African American		37
Afro Caribbean		14
Asian/Pacific Islander		2
White	93	52
Recruitment by Age Group		
Age Group (years)	N	N
18 - 30	6	15

31 - 40	8	15
41 – 50	22	18
51 – 60	26	22
61 – 70	13	13
71 – 80	12	13
Greater than 80	2	3
Continuous variables: Means (standard deviations)		
Age	52.4 (14.7)	50.2 (16.4)
Education	12.7 (2.8)	13.5 (2.0)
TOFHLA Readinga	42.6 (8.3)	46.0 (4.4)
TOFHLA Numeracya	43.7 (6.2)	47.9 (2.8)
REALM	N/Aa	62.6 (6.6)
SAHLSA	45.8 (3.6)	N/Aa
Hospitalb	.66 (.89)	.35 (.76)
Formsb	1.82 (1.20)	2.4 (.94)
Infob	.65 (.95)	.55 (.92)
aReading measures were only administered to participants in Phase 2. The REALM was only administered to English speakers, and the SAHLSA was only administered to Spanish speakers		

bHospital = Chew et al. (2008) self-report screening questions asking whether the participant needs help reading hospital materials, 0 = "never," while 4 = "always"; Forms = Confident in filling out medical forms, 0 = "Not at all," to 3 = "Quite a bit"; Info = Difficulty in understanding written medical information, 0 = "Never," 3 = "Always"

Table 3. Scale descriptions, Cronbach's alpha, and examples

Scale	Examples
General Health Literacy (HL): The ability to read and complete mental operations on health care information, including identify relevant information in prose, documents, and figures (39 items). Cronbach's α for Spanish speakers = 0.81; for English = 0.84; for entire sample = 0.84.	Prose: After reading instructions for laboratory test preparation, correctly identify appointment time. Document: Correctly identify fields in an insurance form; Use an electronic device on a Web page to calculate body mass index.
Numeracy (NUM): The application of quantitative skills including arithmetic operations and appraisal of relations among numeric concepts such as ratios and percentages (24 items). Cronbach's α for Spanish speakers = 0.83; for English = 0.82; for entire sample = 0.84.	Quantitative: Correctly identify meaning of terms related to probability; Correctly identify number of grams of fat consumed in a meal based on values in a table.
Conceptual Knowledge (Experimental Scale; FACT): Demonstrate understanding of specific concepts related to health care (15 items). Cronbach's α for Spanish speakers = 0.58; for English = 0.72; for entire sample = 0.67.	Correctly identify the organ treated by a medical specialist such as a cardiologist

Listening Comprehension (Experimental Scale; LIS): The ability to acquire and remember information presented orally (13 items). Cronbach's α for Spanish speakers = 0.56; for English = 0.60; for entire sample = 0.58.	After viewing a video of a clinician giving information about participation in a clinical research study, correctly identify treatment alternatives.

Table 4. Scale intercorrelations and correlations of the new measure with other measures of health literacy

	HL	NUMa	FACTa	LISa	TOFHLA Reading
HL	1.00	.99**	.67**	.80**	.62**
NUM		1.00	.67**	.77**	.62**
FACT			1.00	.81**	.42**
LIS				1.00	.53**
TOFHLA Reading					1.00
TOFHLA Numeracy					
REALMb					
SAHLSAb					
Hospitalc					
Formsc					
Infoc					

*Correlation is significant at the 0.05 level (2-tailed);
**Correlation is significant at the 0.01 level (2-tailed).
aSome items on NUM, FACT, and LIS were also included in the HL scale, resulting in higher scale intercorrelations.
bThe REALM was only administered to English speakers, and the SAHLSA was only administered to Spanish speakers
cHospital = Need help reading hospital materials;
Forms = Confident in filling out medical forms;
Info= Difficulty in understanding written medical information

TOFHLA Numeracy	REALM	SAHLSA	Hospital	Forms	Info
.34**	.46**	.48**	-.15*	.38**	-.24**
.35**	.48**	.46**	-.16*	.38**	-.24**
.26**	.44**	.56**	-.11	.28**	-.19*
.20**	.34**	.62**	-.05	.32**	-.17*
.29**	.69**	.57**	-.13	.40**	-.25**
1.00	.24*	.17	-.14	.16*	-.12
	1.00	n/ab	-.28**	.23*	-.23*
		1.00	.10	.16	-.25*
			1.00	-.29**	.34**
				1.00	-.31**
					1.00

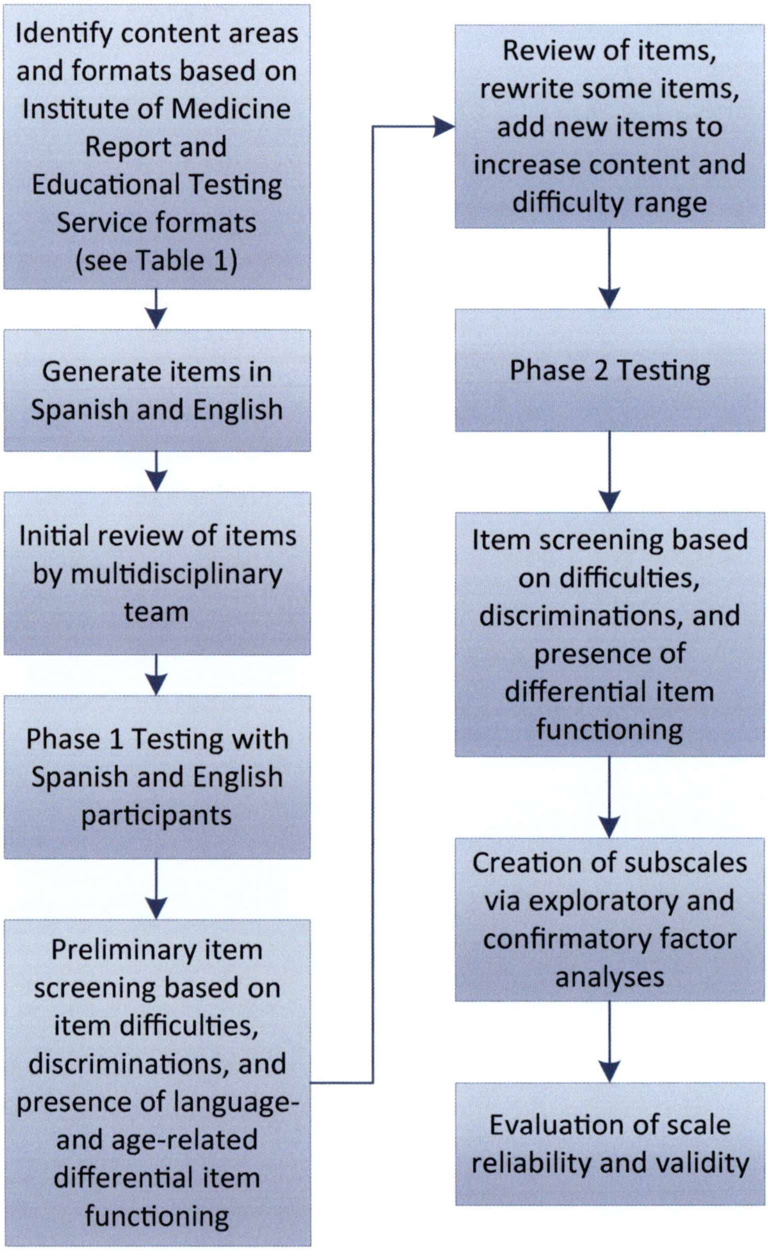

Figure Caption. Item development and testing process

II Validity

This is a copy of a manuscript published in Patient Education and Counseling in 2014. Bibliographic details are available at:
http://www.ncbi.nlm.nih.gov/pubmed/24856447

Quality of Life, Health Status, and Health Service Utilization Related to a New Measure of Health Literacy FLIGHT/VIDAS

Raymond L Ownby1
Amarilis Acevedo2
Robin J. Jacobs1
Joshua Caballero3
Drenna Waldrop-Valverde4

1Department of Psychiatry and Behavioral Medicine, Nova Southeastern University, Fort Lauderdale, FL, USA
2Center for Psychological Studies, Nova Southeastern University, Fort Lauderdale, FL, USA
3College of Pharmacy, Department of Pharmacy Practice, Nova Southeastern University, Fort Lauderdale, FL, USA
4Nell Hodgson Woodruff School of Nursing, Emory University, Atlanta, GA, USA

Corresponding author at: Dr. Ownby, Room 1477, 3200 South University Drive, Fort Lauderdale FL 33314 USA. E-mail: ro71@nova.edu; Voice: +1-954-262-1481.

Supported by grant R01HL096578 from the National Heart, Lung, and Blood Institute to Dr. Ownby.

ABSTRACT
Objective: Researchers have identified significant limitations in some currently-used measures of health literacy. The purpose of this paper is to present data on the relation of health-related quality of life, health status, and health service utilization to performance on a new measure of health literacy in a nonpatient population.
Methods: The new measure was administered to 475 English- and Spanish-speaking community-dwelling volunteers along with existing measures of health literacy and assessments of health-related quality of life, health status, and healthcare service utilization. Relations among measures were assessed via correlations and health status and utilization was tested across levels of health literacy using ANCOVA models.
Results: The new health literacy measure is significantly related to existing measures of health literacy as well as to participants' health-related quality of life. Persons with lower levels of health literacy reported more health conditions, more frequent physical symptoms, and greater healthcare service utilization.
Conclusion: The new measure of health literacy is valid and shows relations to measures of conceptually-related constructs such as quality of life and health behaviors.
Practice Implications: FLIGHT/VIDAS may be useful to researchers and clinicians interested in a computer administered and scored measure of health literacy.

RUNNING HEAD: FLIGHT/VIDAS
KEYWORDS: Health literacy, quality of life, healthcare service utilization, FLIGHT/VIDAS

1. Introduction

Health literacy has been defined as a person's ability to obtain and use health information to make decisions.1 Research shows that health literacy is related to health indicators that include self-reported health, daily functioning, risk for hospitalization and death, and use of healthcare services.2;3 4;5 The observed relations between health literacy and important indicators of health status have led investigators to develop interventions to improve health literacy6;7 in the hope that they may be effective in improving patient health and address race- and ethnicity related health disparities. 8;9 In order to evaluate intervention effectiveness and provide a means to evaluate health literacy as a construct it is necessary to measure it.

Several measures of health literacy have been developed, and each has strengths and weaknesses. Perhaps the most widely-used measure of health literacy is the Test of Functional Health Literacy in Adults.10 The TOFHLA samples a person's performance in reading comprehension as well as in performing simple tasks requiring number skills. The TOFHLA must be administered and scored by a clinician and in general takes 30 minutes. The time required thus limits the TOFHLA's use. The Rapid Estimate of Adult Literacy in Medicine (REALM)11 asks that patients read aloud a list of health-related words. It requires less time to complete than the TOFHLA, but doesn't evaluate whether the patient understands what he or she reads or numeracy skills. The Newest Vital Sign,12 on the other hand, consists of brief questions about a food nutrition label. It is short and easy to administer and score, but assesses only a very small range of health literacy skills.

While measures are thus available, they have also been criticized for other reasons.13-16 Most sample a very limited set of health literacy skills and were developed on small and homogeneous groups of clinic patients rather than the general population.15 Spanish and English versions of several measures are available but it is not clear that they measure the same construct in both languages or are equivalent in difficulty so that their scores can be meaningfully compared. For example, the Spanish and English versions of the TOHFLA Reading subscale are based on the same text passages but require responses to different elements in those passages. Response format may also be an issue, as the cloze procedure used in the TOFHLA reading subtest may be differentially more difficult for older compared to younger persons.17 A final problem with existing measures is that most show pronounced ceiling effects (many persons obtain perfect or near-perfect scores) when administered to groups in the general population. Perhaps reflecting that most were developed with convenience samples of persons at clinics, they function well as screening tools to detect persons with low health literacy. These measures may not work as well to evaluate health literacy in other groups.

A health literacy test that addresses these issues is clearly needed. In addition, a measure that is computer-administered and scored would make assessment of patient and research participant health literacy more easily accessible. Such a measure could be integrated into an electronic health record, automating the process of assessment and interpretation by providing data directly to providers and researchers. This information could in turn be used to provide automated tailoring of information to patients' level of health literacy. This may be an effective strategy to reduce race- and ethnicity-related health disparities.18

A key issue in the development of any new measure is its validity. Standard approaches to validity for new measures of a construct usually center on demonstrating a new measure's relation to existing measures of the same construct (concurrent validity), its ability to predict something in the future (predictive validity), the extent to which the measure represents a coherent or logical concept (construct validity) and the extent to which the items making up the measure have a clear relation to the concept they are believed to measure (content validity). Demonstration of a relation to existing measures of the construct health literacy is a necessary first step in showing that a new test is at least measuring something previously demonstrated to be important. This demonstration is thus key in linking the new test to existing research. In this paper we argue that a useful measure of health literacy should also be related to things that are meaningful to health care consumers as well as in relation to the healthcare system itself. In the project described here, we assessed participants' health-related quality of life, health status by self-report of symptoms and diagnoses, and use of healthcare services such as doctor visits and medications.

The purpose of this paper is to report the relations of a newly-developed computer administered and scored measure of health literacy to existing measures as well as health-related quality of life, health status, and health service utilization. The new measure has been developed in both English and Spanish; the English project is named Fostering Literacy for Good Health Today (FLIGHT) and the Spanish is Vive Desarollando Amplia Salud (VIDAS).

2. Methods

2.1 Overview of initial development

This section provides an overview of the initial development of FLIGHT/VIDAS. Development procedures and analyses establishing the construct validity of FLIGHT/VIDAS have been described in detail in a previous publication19 and are only summarized here. In Phase I of the project, items for the new measure were developed to assess a wide range of healthcare related content, based on the goals of health literacy outlined in the 2004 Institute of Medicine report on health literacy (Table 2-1, p. 42).1 By creating items related to these goals (promote health, understand information, use information, navigate the healthcare system, participate in encounters, give informed consent, and advocate for rights) in three literacy formats (prose, document, quantitative) an initial group of more than 225 questions was created. Items in the measure assess a wide variety of competencies, including information search, critical evaluation of information and strategies for health promotion in addition to content similar to that of existing measures, such as understanding how to take medications or diseases.

These were then pilot tested with community-dwelling older and younger individuals in both English (n = 74) and Spanish (n = 72). The items were screened for equivalent functioning in older and younger persons and in both languages using nonparametric item response theory methods in order to screen items for equivalent function in both languages. A procedure was developed and implemented to evaluate Spanish speakers' competence in both English and Spanish to determine in which language they would complete the study. This was done because other researchers have shown that Spanish speakers who state that they are fluent in English may be at a significant disadvantage compared to native English speakers on measures of health literacy.20

During phase II of the project a reduced group of 98 items was administered to community-dwelling individuals from a wide range of ages, educational backgrounds, and across genders and race/ethnicity groups. Participants also completed a battery of measures intended to allow the measure's validation not only in relation to other tests of health literacy but also to variables judged clinically meaningful. This battery thus included existing measures of health literacy and measures of health-related quality of life, health status and health service utilization.

In a previous publication we reported on the preliminary evaluation of the measure's reliability and validity with an interim sample of 198 participants .21 We concluded that, given the material assessed by the items of FLIGHT/VIDAS, the measure has clear content validity. In the previous publication we also described exploratory and confirmatory factor analyses that established the construct validity of the measure as representing four scales, general health literacy, numeracy, literacy, and conceptual knowledge. Data presented here are for the final sample of 475 participants.

2.2 Sample

Participants were recruited via flyers, presentations at community organizations, and by recruitment from previous studies. Purposive sampling focused on recruiting groups of Spanish- and English-speaking participants in the age ranges 18-30; 31-40; 41-50; 51-60; 61-70; 71-80; and 81 years and older. Recruitment was targeted to various socioeconomic, occupational, and educational backgrounds (e.g., ranging from grade school to doctoral-level graduate education) and, in the case of Spanish-speaking participants, to a range of national origins (Central and South America as well as Mexico and the US). This strategy allowed the recruitment of a diverse group of nonpatients so that preliminary norms for the new measure can be created. Participants were compensated for their participation.

2.3 Measures

As well as the new health literacy scale, participants completed a battery of existing measures (TOFHLA in English or Spanish; REALM or SAHL-SA, and the self-report questions developed by Chew et al.22). Using a procedure modified from the MIDUS study,23 they provided information on their health status as the number and frequency of common physical symptoms they experienced (e.g., how often they had a headache) and the number of conditions they reported (e.g., heart disease, lung disease, cancer).

Health-related quality of life was assessed with the Rand Medical Outcomes Study Short Form-36 (SF-36),[24] and mood with the Center for Epidemiological Studies Depression Scale (CES-D).[25] The EQ-5D is a widely-used health utility index that can be derived from SF-36 scales.[26] It provides a single general measure of health status that can be used in economic analyses and to track the impact of healthcare interventions, and has been shown to be useful in a number of conditions.[27-32]

We asked participants how often they saw a physician or other provider and whether they took medications for health conditions such as hypertension or pain. When participants reported that they took medications, they were asked about how frequently they took them (e.g., every day for antihypertensives vs. occasional use of medication for headache). These measures were selected to allow the evaluation of the relation of the new measure to existing tests of health literacy to establish its concurrent validity with standard and widely-accepted measures. Other assessments (quality of life, health status, and health service utilization) were included to establish the new measure's relation to clinically relevant variables that are not directly related to reading or education.

2.4 Data Analyses

Previous analyses[19] showed that FLIGHT/VIDAS has four scales: general health literacy (HL), numeracy (NUM), conceptual knowledge (FACT) and listening (LIS). Cronbach's alpha was calculated for the scales of FLIGHT/VIDAS. Correlations of the FLIGHT/VIDAS scales with the TOFHLA, REALM, SAHLSA, and self-report questions were calculated to assess concurrent validity. We evaluated the relation of various levels of health literacy for health status, physician visits and medication use by defining groups with low, medium, and high levels of health literacy on the FLIGHT/VIDAS HL scale. Between-group differences were then assessed via analysis of variance (ANOVA).

All study procedures were completed under a protocol approved by the Institutional Review Board of Nova Southeastern University.

3. RESULTS

3.1 Descriptive data

Demographic data for participants (236 English- and 239 Spanish-speaking participants) are presented in Table 1. Spanish-speaking participants described their racial background as white or mixed race, consistent with findings from the US Census33 while English-speaking participants were African American, Afro Caribbean, white, and Asian. Consistent with our sampling strategy, the average age of our participants is approximately 50, and the average level of education was equivalent to having completed high school. Our actual recruitment by target age groups is also included in this table. Table 2 presents descriptive statistics for the measures used to establish the concurrent validity of FLIGHT/VIDAS.

Insert Tables 1 & 2 about here

3.2 Reliability

Cronbach's alphas for the scales of FLIGHT/VIDAS were 0.87 for HL for the combined sample (0.85 for English and 0.87 for Spanish speakers), 0.88 for NUM (0.87 for English and 0.85 for Spanish), 0.69 for FACT (0.74 for English and 0.60 for Spanish), and 0.55 for LIS (0.63 for English and 0.51 for Spanish). Consistent with our previous report on the reliabilities of the FACT and LIS scales,19 we suggest that they be used for research purposes only.

3.3 Concurrent validity.

Correlations of the FLIGHT/VIDAS scales with other measures of health literacy are presented in Table 3. It can be seen that even though FLIGHT/VIDAS was developed with a much broader range of content and uses a different response format, its scales are still significantly correlated with other tests of health literacy. Correlations of the FLIGHT/VIDAS scales with established measures of health literacy are similar to those among the established measures themselves.

Insert Table 3 about here

Correlations of FLIGHT/VIDAS with a measure of health-related quality of life and health utility (SF-36 scales and the EQ-5D) are presented in Table 4. This table includes participants' total TOFHLA score to allow comparisons. The FLIGHT/VIDAS scales were correlated at low to moderate34 levels with several SF-36 scales, including General Health, Physical Functioning, Social Functioning, and Emotional Wellbeing. All scales of

FLIGHT/VIDAS were significantly correlated with the health utility index, the EQ-5D.

Insert Table 4 about here

3.4 Range of scores

Most available measures of health literacy show pronounced ceiling effects when used in the general population, limiting their use in evaluating health literacy in nonpatients groups. A specific focus of FLIGHT/VIDAS development was to ensure that items with difficulties of sufficient difficulty were created that would be challenging even for well-educated participants. Figure 1 presents a histogram of HL scale scores for English and Spanish-speaking participants. It can be seen that the range of scores on HL is substantial and includes a number of cases at the lower and higher ends of the range. Scores on HL ranged from 7 to 39 (of 40), on NUM from 0 to 24 (of 24), FACT from 0 to 14 (of 14), and LIS from 3 to 12 (of 12). Ranges for the two language groups were similar.

Insert Figure 1 about here

3.5 Levels of health literacy, health status, and service utilization

Analysis of covariance (ANCOVA) models assessed differences health status and utilization variables across groups defined by scores on the HL scale of FLIGHT/VIDAS. Models included age, gender, race, education, and language as covariates in order to take these possible confounders into account. Groups were established at the cut points for the 33rd and 66th percentile of scores, resulting in a group with low (n = 131), intermediate (n = 134), and high (n = 157) levels of health literacy. ANCOVA models are presented in Table 5. Those with the highest levels of health literacy reported fewer conditions and symptoms, less frequent use of medications and fewer doctor visits.

4. Discussion and Conclusion

4.1 Discussion

This paper reports on the relation of a new measure of health literacy, FLIGHT/VIDAS, to other measures of health literacy and to a measure of health-related quality of life. We also evaluated the relation of level of health literacy as assessed by the scale to health status and health care service utilization. Analyses show that FLIGHT/VIDAS scales are correlated significantly with established measures of health literacy and a well-known measure of health-related quality of life. Persons with varying levels of health literacy as assessed by the FLIGHT/VIDAS show significant differences in health status and health service utilization.

We had previously provided a preliminary report of the relations of the FLIGHT/VIDAS scales to other measures with analyses based on a much smaller interim sample.19 This paper supplements this earlier report with analyses using the final full sample of participants. The core scales (HL and NUM) of FLIGHT/VIDAS have excellent reliability and significant correlations with established tests of health literacy and with participant self-report of difficulties in reading health-related materials, showing that it is likely to be a valid measure of health literacy. Their range of scores shows that the scales may be useful across a number of ability levels, potentially making FLIGHT/VIDAS more useful for research on health literacy in the general population than other measure that show marked ceiling effects.

The purpose of this paper has also been to go beyond solely demonstrating the new measure's relation to established scales and to relate performance on it to meaningful clinical status and utilization variables such as health-related quality of life, use of healthcare services, and health utility. Results show that performance on FLIGHT/VIDAS is related in small to moderately large ways to multiple aspects of health related quality of life. Results show that participants with the highest levels of health literacy report fewer health conditions, fewer and less frequent symptoms, less medication use and fewer doctor visits.

The guiding principles in creating FLIGHT/VIDAS were to create a new measure that addressed limitations of existing measures and was computer administered and scored. One important limitation has been that some measures have not been demonstrated to have relations to variables in addition to other measures of health literacy. Exceptions include the TOFHLA, which has been related to cognitive function, quality of life, and health utilization. The TOFHLA, however, focuses on a narrow range of content, relies on the cloze procedure to assess reading comprehension, and must be hand administered and scored. While it is effective for detecting persons with low health literacy it suffers from substantial ceiling effects when used in other populations. FLIGHT/VIDAS addresses these issues. It includes diverse content ranging from reading pill bottle labels to understanding health promotion messages. It does not rely on the cloze procedure which may be more difficult for older compared to younger persons.17 It can be administered and scored with little or no clinician intervention, and has a wide range of scores in a normal population. Data presented here demonstrate that FLIGHT/VIDAS performance is related to meaningful variables such as health-related quality of life and use of health services suggesting that it may be a useful addition to current measures in clinical practice and in research. Given its range of health-related content and wide range of scores in the general population, FLIGHT/VIDAS may be useful in research studies examining the impact of individuals' health literacy on the interactions with organizations that themselves have varying levels of health literacy35;36 and in better understanding health literacy as a social construct.16;37

4.2 Conclusion

The new measure of health literacy, FLIGHT/VIDAS, is computer-administered and scored and shows evidence of excellent reliability and significant relations to better-established measures of health literacy. It includes content not only related to tasks such as taking medications or understanding disease but also to information search, health promotion activities, and critical evaluation of health information. Given its potential broader use in nonclinical populations, it may be a useful addition to research on health literacy. As it is computer administered and scored, it may also be a useful addition to clinical practice, making information on patients' health literacy more readily available for use by clinicians. We plan to support its dissemination by making it available for use online and by providing a standard manual for administration that will include preliminary norms.

4.3 Practice Implications

FLIGHT/VIDAS may be a useful addition to existing measures of health literacy. It addresses several limitations of other tests of health literacy and can be administered in an automated fashion. A disadvantage of the measure is that it requires computer equipment for use. Advantages include the broad content assessed, the wide range of scores in the general population, its clear relation not only to existing measures but also to clinically meaningful health status and utilization, and its availability in English and Spanish. FLIGHT/VIDAS may thus be useful for research and clinical practice in contexts in which its can be administered and its length is not prohibitive. It may be especially advantageous for research on health literacy in the general population and among persons with average to above average educational backgrounds where existing tests show ceiling effects.

DISCLOSURES

All authors state that they have no conflicts of interest to disclose.

ACKNOWLEDGEMENT

The study described in this paper was supported by grant R01HL096578 to Dr. Ownby from the National Heart, Lung, and Blood Institute.

Table 1. Description of participants		
	English (N = 236)	Spanish (N = 239)
Gender M/F	94 (40%) / 142 (60%)	94 (39%) / 145 (61%)
Hispanic	24	239
African American	86	0
Afro Caribbean	26	0
Asian/Pacific Islander	2	0
Mixed Race	0	2
White	122	237
Participants' Age Group		
Age Group (years)	N	N
18 - 30	33	26
31 - 40	35	30
41 – 50	35	55
51 – 60	40	34
61 – 70	40	34
71 – 80	38	35
Greater than 80	13	8
Means (standard deviations)		
Age	51.9 (18.4)	51.7 (16.5)
Education	13.2 (2.4)	11.7 (3.3)
Income	$31,894 ($24,471)	$26,088 ($21,752)

Table 2. Descriptive statistics for validity measures

	Mean (SD)			T (df)	p
	English	Spanish	t	df	p
TOFHLA Readinga	45.7 (5.5)	42.8 (9.5)	5.45	472	< .001
TOFHLA Numeracya	47.4 (3.7)	42.6 (6.7)	9.63	473	< .001
TOFHLA Total	93.0 (8.0)	84.4 (14.1)	8.28	472	< .001
REALM	62.1 (8.0)	N/Aa			
SAHLSA	N/Aa	45.1 (4.5)			
Hospitalb	.31 (.73)	.73 (1.04)	-4.97	459	< .001
Formsb	2.5 (.93)	2.0 (1.12)	4.69	460	< .001
Infob	.48 (.85)	.79 (1.09)	-3.29	456	< .001
SF Phys Func	77.3 (25.9)	83.9 (21.3)	-2.98	450	.003
SF Limit Phys Func	23.1 (37.3)	13.3 (29.2)	3.13	455	.002
SF Limit Emot Probs	20.1 (34.3)	16.6 (33.7)	1.09	451	.27
SF Energy/Fatigue	64.3 (21.2)	72.7 (18.8)	-4.55	458	< .001
SF Emotional Wellbeing	80.6 (16.6)	77.0 (18.2)	2.22	457	.03
SF Social Function	84.4 (20.9)	84.7 (19.3)	.11	456	.91
SF Pain	72.9 (25.0)	78.4 (22.0)	-2.52	459	.01
SF General Health	70.9 (18.9)	73.4 (17.5)	-1.42	451	.16
Physical Symptoms	14.7 (9.4)	11.7 (9.4)	3.19	405	.002
Health Conditions	3.3 (3.2)	2.6 (3.1)	2.48	456	.01
Medications	1.4 (1.5)	1.3 (1.5)	.80	462	.42

Table 4. Correlations of health literacy measures with SF-36 and EQ-5D

	HL	NUM	FACT	LIS	TOF-HLA Total	SF Phys Func	SF Limit Phys Func
HL	1.00	.82**	.72**	.65**	.69**	.27**	-0.08
NUM		1.00	.53**	.57**	.63**	.24**	-0.07
FACT			1.00	.42**	.46**	0.08	0.01
LIS				1.00	.53**	.21**	-0.07
TOFHLA Total					1.00	.25**	-0.09
SF Phys Func						1.00	-.63**
SF Limit Phys Func							1.00
SF Limit Emot Probls							
SF Energy/ Fatigue							
SF Emotional Wellbeing							
SF Social Function							

SF Limit Emot Probls	SF Energy/ Fatigue	SF Emo-tional Wellbe-ing	SF Social Function	SF Pain	SF General Health	EQ 5D
-.11*	0.07	.22**	.17**	.12**	.14**	.26**
-0.08	0.01	.15**	.18**	.13**	.10*	.23**
-0.09	0.06	.18**	.13**	0.05	.11*	.11*
-.11*	0.03	.14**	.13**	0.09	0.04	.18**
-0.07	0.02	.14**	.10*	0.05	.13**	.19**
-.31**	.45**	.25**	.39**	.61**	.45**	.87**
.31**	-.46**	-.29**	-.49**	-.62**	-.43**	-.71**
1.00	-.48**	-.61**	-.61**	-.34**	-.37**	-.49**
	1.00	.64**	.59**	.53**	.63**	.64**
		1.00	.65**	.34**	.47**	.56**
			1.00	.50**	.51**	.67**

Table 5. Utilization for health literacy groups						
	Level of Health Literacy					
Variable	Low	Interme-diate	High	df	F	p
Conditions	3.6 (3.4)	2.8 (2.9)	2.4 (2.4)	2, 414	3.01	0.050
Symptoms	15.5 (10.3)	13.4 (9.6)	10.1 (8.0)a	2, 370	6.64	0.001
Medications	1.7 (1.7)	1.3 (1.6)	1.0 (1.2)a	2, 420	3.78	0.02
Doctor Visits	11.5 (17.9)	10.8 (19.6)	7.0 (7.3)b	2, 381	3.32	0.04
aSignificantly different from values for low and intermediate groups, p < 0.05						
bSignificantly different from value for intermediate group, p < 0.05.						

III ASK Model

This is a copy of a manuscript that appeared in *Patient Education and Counseling.* The definitive version of this manuscript appears on the publisher's web site. Bibliographic information for this paper can be found at:

http://www.ncbi.nlm.nih.gov/pubmed/24637163

And a copy of the final manuscript is available for download at:

http://www.ncbi.nlm.nih.gov/pmc/articles/PMC4040019/

Abilities, Skills and Knowledge in Measures of Health Literacy

Raymond L Ownby[1]

Amarilis Acevedo[2]

Drenna Waldrop-Valverde[3]

Robin J Jacobs[1]

Joshua Caballero[4]

[1]Department of Psychiatry and Behavioral Medicine, Nova Southeastern University, Fort Lauderdale FL

2Center for Psychological Studies, Nova Southeastern University, Fort Lauderdale, FL

3Nell Hodgson Woodruff School of Nursing, Emory University, Atlanta, GA

4College of Pharmacy, Department of Pharmacy Practice, Nova Southeastern University, Fort Lauderdale, FL

Correspondence to: Dr. Ownby, Room 1477, 3200 South University Drive, Fort Lauderdale, FL 33314. E-mail: ro71@nova.edu; Voice: +1-954-262-1481

Abstract

Objective: Health literacy has been recognized as an important factor in patients' health status and outcomes, but the relative contribution of demographic variables, cognitive abilities, academic skills, and health knowledge to performance on tests of health literacy has not been as extensively explored. The purpose of this paper is to propose a model of health literacy as a composite of cognitive abilities, academic skills, and health knowledge (ASK model) and test its relation to measures of health literacy in a model that first takes demographic variables into account.

Methods: A battery of cognitive, academic achievement, health knowledge and health literacy measures was administered to 359 Spanish- and English-speaking community-dwelling volunteers. The relations of health literacy tests to the model were evaluated using regression models.

Results: Each health literacy test was related to elements of the model but variability existed across measures.

Conclusion: Analyses partially support the ASK model defining health literacy as a composite of abilities, skills, and knowledge, although the relations of commonly-used health literacy measures to each element of the model varied widely.

Practice implications: Results suggest that clinicians and researchers should be aware of the abilities and skills assessed by health literacy measures when choosing a measure.

200 words

Abilities, Skills and Knowledge in Measures of Health Literacy

1. Introduction

Health literacy, defined as an individual's ability to obtain and use health information to make choices about health care, is related to patients' health [1;2], health status, service utilization, self-care behaviors, and even risk for death [2;3] and has been tied to race- and ethnicity-related disparities.[4-6]. In spite of the large amount of research on it, important questions about health literacy remain, such as how it can most effectively be defined to facilitate measurement and develop effective interventions. In most studies, health literacy has been assessed as patient performance on a test of health literacy, but each of the commonly-used measures evaluates health literacy in a different way. In some instances, health literacy is defined as reading comprehension (the Reading subtest of Test of Functional Health Literacy in Adults, or TOFHLA [7]), sight-word reading (the Rapid Estimate of Adult Literacy in Medicine, or REALM [8]), calculation (the Numeracy subtest of the TOFHLA), or identifying synonyms (the Short Assessment of Health Literacy for Spanish Adults, or SAHLSA [9]). Each of these strategies assesses something related to health literacy, but their diversity leaves open the question of what each has in common with the "social construct of health literacy." [10]

Each measure samples different content, uses different response formats, and has been developed on different populations [11]. The TOFHLA, for example, evaluates reading comprehension by asking a person to supply words eliminated from the text (the cloze procedure), while its numeracy scale asks that he or she explain how to take medications. The REALM requires the person to correctly read aloud words related to healthcare. The need for a similar measure for Spanish speakers led to the development of the SAHLSA, but the low frequency of orthographically-irregular words in Spanish meant that it was necessary to develop a different response format. The SAHLSA asks the person tested to view a stimulus word on a card and choose which of two other words is most similar in meaning.

Performance on these measures requires reading and health knowledge, and several, especially the TOFHLA subtests, also require reasoning, problem solving and numeracy [12]. The variety of contents and formats, however, suggests that the abilities, skills, and knowledge required for successful performance on each are different [13;14]. Griffin et al., for example, showed substantial differences in which patients were identified as having limited health literacy by different measures [15], and similar findings have been reported in other studies [13;16]. Because of this, it was hypothesized that more clearly establishing the relations of widely-used tests of health literacy to other variables might provide a better understand what each measures. It was also hypothesized that a better understanding would also provide a clearer picture of what health literacy is by more clearly delineating its component skills. In this paper, it is hypothesized that the variables most relevant to health literacy are individuals' general cognitive abilities and academic skills, and their health-related knowledge, after their demographic characteristics (race, ethnicity, age, and SES) are taken into account.

1.1 Health literacy and demographic variables

Studies have shown that health literacy is related to age, race, ethnicity, and socioeconomic status. For example, persons older than 65 years of age performed at lower levels on the Health Literacy scale of the National Assessment of Adult Literacy [17]. Blacks and Hispanics have also been shown to perform at lower levels on measures of health literacy. Closely intertwined with other demographic characteristics is socioeconomic status, itself related to health literacy [18]. The finding that English-speaking

Hispanics may be at a disadvantage to non-Hispanics when their health literacy is assessed in English [19] suggests that preferred language may also be a key characteristic. Gender may also be related to performance on tests of health literacy [19].

1.2 Health literacy and cognition

Understanding the relation of tests of health literacy to basic cognitive abilities (or intelligence, often assessed by IQ tests) may be especially important since research has shown that both general intellectual abilities and health literacy are related to health [20-23]. General intellectual ability can be defined as reflecting a person's acquired knowledge and communication ability (crystallized ability) and capacity to reason and solve novel problems (fluid ability) [24-26]. Baker et al. [23] showed that overall performance on the Mini-mental State Exam (MMSE; [27]) was related to S-TOFHLA scores. Levinthal et al. [28] evaluated the relation of demographic and cognitive variables to performance on the S-TOFHLA and found that both were related. Chin et al. [21] found that age, education, basic cognitive abilities, and disease-related knowledge were related to performance on the S-TOHLA and REALM. Others have shown that performance on tests of health literacy is related to various abilities including memory, verbal fluency, reasoning, and general intellectual functioning [22;29;30].

1.3 Health literacy and academic skills

By its very nature, health literacy appears related to academic skills such as reading and mathematics [31-33]. Academic skills can be distinguished from basic cognitive abilities by their acquisition via formal instruction during schooling. While basic cognitive abilities are thought to be stable over time [34], academic skills such as reading, writing, and arithmetic are amenable to change through formal interventions well into adult life [35]. While it is important to distinguish between general reading skills and health literacy [36;37], the correlation between patients' performance on measures of academic skills and health literacy has been presented as evidence of the measures' validity [38;39].

1.4 Health literacy and health knowledge

In addition to demographics, cognitive abilities and academic skills, health knowledge is related both to performance on tests of health literacy and health. Disease-specific knowledge, for example, has been linked to health literacy in diabetes [40], hypertension [21;41], HIV infection [42], asthma, and congestive heart failure [41].

1.5 Synthesis: The ASK model

These studies illustrate the diverse influences affecting performance on tests of health literacy. Demographics, cognitive abilities, academic skills, and health knowledge are each related to scores on measures of health literacy. Few studies have included variables from all of these domains, however, and studies that have used variables from multiple domains have shown that variables from one domain may reduce the importance of others. In this paper, it is hypothesized that after taking demographic characteristics into account, each group of variables will define health literacy as a unique entity depending on a person's general intellectual abilities, academic skills and health-related knowledge (ASK).

2. Method

As part of a larger study whose purpose has been to develop a new computer-administered measure of health literacy [43], participants completed a battery of general intellectual, academic skills, and health literacy measures. They were recruited from the community through publicity at various local organizations, distribution of flyers, and referral by persons who had already completed the study.

2.1 Measures

2.1.1 Demographics

Participant age, education, occupation, income, gender, and race were recorded. Principal factor analysis was used to construct a composite index of socioeconomic status based on education, income, and occupational prestige index [44]. The index was constructed to address the limitations of single-indicator measures [45], as single indicators such as education, income, and occupational status are only moderately correlated and only partially represent an individual's status [46]. The index was calculated by including education, occupational prestige, and income in a principal factor analysis [47]. Each indicator's loading on a single factor (0.27, 0.27, and 0.16 for education, occupational status, and income, respectively) provided weights for calculation of factor scores for each participant.

2.1.2 Cognitive Abilities.

Crystallized general cognitive abilities [24;25] were assessed using the Verbal Composite score of the Woodcock-Johnson Psycho-Educational Battery for English speakers and the Woodcock-Muñoz Psycho-Educational Battery for Spanish speakers (WJPEB/WMPEB; [48;49]). These measures tap word knowledge, general information, and verbal reasoning in a series of tasks that yields a single score. Fluid general cognitive abilities were assessed with the Block Design and Matrix Reasoning subtests of the Wechsler Adult Intelligence Scale, Third Edition [50]; the average of these subtests' age-corrected scores yielded an index [24;25].

2.1.3 Academic Skills

Reading and mathematics skills were assessed with the Passage Comprehension and Applied Problems subtests of the WJPEB/WMPEB [48;49]. The Passage Comprehension subtests use items based on one or two sentences to evaluate reading comprehension. The Applied Problems subtests assess mathematics skill through items requiring problem solving as well as calculation.

2.1.4 Health Knowledge

Health knowledge was assessed with a subscale of the new measure developed during the study [43]. Baker commented on the potential usefulness of a brief measure of general health knowledge [33] and As part of our project [43], we developed such a measure. It comprises 15 questions, all of which assess knowledge of a specific fact, such as a disease risk factor or a specific drug treatment for a disease, and do not require substantial reading or numeracy skills, as for example, "Cholesterol is measured with a . . ." Other items assessed a broad range of health-related facts, include the part of the body most commonly treated by a specific medical profession (nephrology), what common over-the-counter medications are used for (aspirin for heart attack), and the meaning of blood lipid indices (e.g., HDL).

The health knowledge scale was developed in two stages. A group of candidate items was first administered to older and younger Spanish or English speaking individuals. Preliminary analyses of item performance in both languages and of item discrimination and difficulty allowed us to choose items for the second phase of the study. In this phase, scale items were administered along with the additional measures as described here. The dimensional structure of the new knowledge scale as well as item difficulties were supported through psychometric analyses [43], although its marginally acceptable internal reliability (Cronbach's alpha = 0.67) limits its use to research.

2.1.4 Health Literacy

All participants completed either the Spanish or English versions of the Test of Functional Health Literacy in Adults (TOFHLA; [7]). English-speakers completed the Rapid Estimate of Adult Literacy in Medicine (REALM [8]), while Spanish speakers completed the Short Assessment of Health Literacy for Spanish-speaking Adults (SAHLSA [9]).

2.2 Analyses

Linear regression models using progressively more complex blocks of variables representing, first, demographics and then the elements of the ASK model were created to assess study hypotheses. Variable blocks after correcting for demographics were evaluated in a logical order from the most general and basic (core intellectual abilities) through the more specific skills acquired early in life (reading or mathematics) to the most specific (health-related knowledge). Models assessed the relative contribution of each element to prediction of each measure. Analyses were completed using SPSS version 21 (Montauk, NY: IBM).

All study procedures were completed under a protocol approved by the Nova Southeastern University Institutional Review Board. Verbal consent was obtained from participants for screening procedures and written informed consent was obtained from all subjects prior to their participation.

3. Results

Descriptive statistics for the sample are presented in Table 1. Our sample intentionally included participants from a wide range of ages (18 to 85) and the mean age for the combined sample was 51.0 years (standard deviation = 16.5). The sample included individuals with a wide range of education (3 to 20 years) with a combined sample mean of 12.9 years (standard deviation = 2.6).

Regression models are presented in Tables 2 to 5. Results for the TOFHLA Reading subtest (Table 2) show that in the model only including demographic variables (Model 1), SES was related to higher scores on the TOFHLA Reading while age, being black, and speaking Spanish were related to lower scores (Model 1 $R2 = 0.19$, $F = [df = 5, 278] = 13.32$, $p < 0.001$). Both crystallized and fluid abilities added to the model's prediction of TOFHLA scores (Model 2 $R2 = 0.41$, F for change = [df = 2, 276] = 49.11, $p < 0.001$), while reading added still further to the model ($R2 = 0.43$, F for change = [df = 1, 275] = 9.86, $p = 0.002$), as did health knowledge ($R2 = 0.44$, F for change = [df = 1, 274] = 8.20, $p = 0.005$).

The model for the TOFHLA Numeracy subtest (Table 3) also showed that SES was positively and Spanish language was inversely related to scores ($R2 = 0.18$, $F = [df = 5, 279] = 12.53$, $p < 0.001$). The addition of general cognitive abilities increased prediction ($R2 = 0.21$, F for change = [df = 2, 277] = 8.36, $p < 0.001$). The addition of math skills did not improve prediction ($R2 = 0.21$, F for change = [df = 1, 276] = 1.60, $p = 0.21$) even though it was related to the Numeracy subscale (Table 3). Addition of health knowledge to the model did not improve prediction ($R2 = 0.22$, F for change = [df = 1, 275] = 3.17, $p = 0.08$).

Separate models for each language group for the TOHFLA are available as supplementary materials to this paper.

The model for English speakers on the REALM is presented in Table 4. In Model 1, female gender was positively and black race was inversely related to scores. ($R2 = 0.17$, F = [df = 4, 134] = 6.62, $p < 0.001$). The addition of general cognitive abilities improved prediction ($R2 = 0.25$, F for change = [df = 2, 132] = 7.88, $p = 0.001$), as did the addition of reading ($R2 = 0.28$, F for change = [df = 1, 131] = 5.03, $p = 0.02$), and knowledge ($R2 = 0.34$, F for change = [df = 1, 130] = 19.77, $p < 0.0001$).

The model for the SAHLSA is presented in Table 5. In Model 1, only SES was associated with better scores although the value for female gender approached statistical significance ($R2 = 0.07$, F model = [df = 3, 142] = 3.42, $p = 0.02$). The addition of crystallized and fluid abilities did not improve prediction ($R2 = 0.10$, F for change = [df = 2, 140] = 2.81, $p = 0.06$) although crystallized abilities were a significant predictor. Neither the addition of academic reading ($R2 = 0.12$ F for change = [df = 1, 139] = 2.51, $p = 0.12$) nor knowledge ($R2 = 0.14$, F for change = [df = 1, 139] = 2.69, $p = 0.10$) increased prediction.

Table 6 presents a summary of the variability (R2) accounted for by each block and the significance of change associated with each. The percentage of variability related to demographic variables was similar for the TOFHLA subtests and the REALM while the SAHLSA was less strongly related to demographic variables. TOFHLA Reading scores were significantly related to cognitive abilities, while scores on the other measures were much less clearly related to cognition. Academic skills provided similar contributions in each model, except for the TOFHLA Numeracy subtest which, while a significant predictor, did not improve overall model prediction. In most models, health knowledge provided a small but significant contribution.

4. Discussion and Conclusion

4.1 Discussion

The purpose of these analyses was to assess how performance on health literacy measures was related to abilities, skills, and knowledge as specified by the ASK model. Results for several measures support the model, especially those for the TOFHLA Reading subscale. Support was less substantial for other measures, but all included at least one model element. Analyses for each measure do not uniformly include model elements, suggesting that important aspects of health literacy as measured by some tests are not captured by the model. The elements of the model are most clearly related to the TOFHLA reading subtest; to the extent that it can be considered a gold standard for health literacy measurement, the ASK model is supported, but further research is needed. These findings provide insight into diverse factors related to performance on health literacy measures and are consistent with the view of health literacy as a unique combination of abilities, skills and knowledge.

Results of these analyses raise an important issue about the use of these measures in research, since most studies have implicitly operationalized "health literacy" as participants' performance one of them. Although researchers in the field of health literacy have acknowledged that it is a complex concept [10;31], and have argued for the evolution of its definition [32], substantial work remains in order to better define what health literacy is and how it can be distinguished from closely related concepts such as general literacy, education, and mathematics skills. Clear differences exist in these measures, and it may be difficult to generalize about the concept of health literacy from studies that use different measures. Results thus confirm and extend others' observations of the diverse relations of health literacy measures to other abilities and skills [13;14;16] and support the recommendation of Haun et al. [13] that researchers and clinicians be alert to differences among measures.

Examination of groups of predictors in sequential blocks also assists in interpretation of findings from other studies of race- and language-related differences in health literacy. Results for Model 1 (demographic variables only) across measures revealed differences in performance on health literacy measures related to age, SES, race, and language; the impact of these factors was reduced or eliminated when cognitive abilities, academic skills, and health knowledge were included in models. For example, while in Model 1 for the TOFHLA Reading subscale blacks performed at lower levels compared to whites, race was no longer a significant predictor when abilities, skills and health knowledge were taken into account (Model 4 in Table 2). This might imply that a portion of the often-observed relation of demographic variables to health literacy may reflect individuals' history of educational opportunities [51] and that race- or ethnicity-related differences in health literacy could be addressed through educational interventions [6;52-56].

An important aspect of the TOFHLA analyses presented here is the use of a combined sample that had been evaluated in either Spanish or English. We chose this combined sample strategy as it provided the opportunity to understand the impact of ASK model variables while taking language into account. The combined sample also conferred the benefit of increased statistical power to detect relationships while evaluating the relation of SES, age, cognitive abilities, academic skills, and health knowledge on ethnicity-related differences in performance on health literacy measures. Similar to our findings on the reduced relation of race to health literacy when other variables are controlled, these analyses show that the relation of language was reduced when ability, skills, and knowledge were included in regression models. It should be noted, however, that language-related differences in performance on the TOFHLA subtests may reflect differences in the measures as well as difference in the persons assessed, since to the best of our knowledge no study has demonstrated that the Spanish and English versions of the TOFHLA, while similar in content, are psychometrically equivalent.

Another noteworthy result related to the TOFHLA was our failure to find a relation of its Numeracy scale to general intellectual abilities or knowledge (although fluid abilities and knowledge approached significance as predictors). Examination of the content of the TOFHLA Numeracy scale shows that it includes a number of task demands beyond numeracy, including auditory attention and listening skills (most questions are presented orally even if supported by props such as pill bottles and information cards), visual attention (detecting specific information on pill bottle labels), and reasoning (deciding who should be included in determining the number of members in a household). It may be that this scale assesses a construct that is not included in the ASK model, or conversely, that its independent relation to other measures is weak due to its diverse content and brevity. Few studies have investigated its psychometric properties independent of the full TOHFLA, and we note that many investigators have chosen to use the S-TOHFLA [57], which reduces the number of numeracy items to four. A clearer explanation of this finding must await additional study.

Other studies have reported regression models and the variability accounted for by similar groups of variables, though none has included all of the domains reported on here. Levinthal et al. [28] included demographics and cognitive variables in predicting the S-TOFHLA; their model accounted for 49% of the variability scores. Chin et al. also included demographic and cognitive variables in predicting the S-TOFHLA and the REALM. Their models accounted for 32% of the variability in REALM scores and 42% of S-TOFHLA scores. Yost et al. report a model included demographic and several brief cognitive measures predicting scores on the computer-administered Health LiTT [30]; it accounted for 27% of its variability. The values we report for the TOFHLA Reading and the REALM are thus similar to those found by other investigators, but also demonstrate the importance of reading skills and health knowledge.

Limitations of our study should be acknowledged and include the nature of our sample. Our participants were drawn from the community rather than from groups of patients in health care organizations as has been true of many other studies [11]. Although in some ways a strength, our sample, as is common in volunteer research, has higher levels of education than the general population. Because of our strategy of sampling across age groups, it included a wider age range than in most other studies. It is possible that our findings might not be the same in groups with a lower education levels, older persons, or in persons seeking medical care. It should be noted that education is included in the SES index used so that differences related to education are accounted for in regression models. It may also be noted that although the mean level of education of our participants is high, the sample included a wide range of educational attainment (as low as three years to doctoral-level), potentially reducing this issue's impact. Conversely, as the sample includes a wide range of age and educational levels and was recruited from the community, these results may be more broadly generalizable to the general population.

4.2 Conclusion

These analyses suggest that the ASK model may be useful in understanding individuals' performance on measures of health literacy. They highlight the impact of demographic characteristics and general cognitive abilities as determinants of performance on measures of health literacy and extend our understanding of the role of academic skills and health knowledge in health literacy. To the extent that health literacy measures are used to operationally define it, then results can be interpreted as support for the definition of health literacy as a unique combination of abilities, skills, and knowledge. Results thus provide support for the ASK model and suggest it might be a helpful framework within which to understand health literacy and to distinguish it from general cognitive ability or literacy alone.

4.3 Practice Implications

Differences in predictors among the measures highlight the heterogeneity of what they measure. While the TOFHLA Reading Comprehension scale was clearly associated with both crystallized and fluid abilities as well as academic reading skills and conceptual knowledge, in the model including all predictors the SAHLSA was not clearly associated with any. Our findings thus confirm and extend those of others who have noted the diverse number of abilities and skills assessed by measures of health literacy and the various ways in which they are related [13;14;16]. It is suggested that practitioners be aware of this variability in choosing a health literacy test since it is clear that different tests of health literacy measure different things. The relations of the TOFHLA Numeracy subtest and the SAHLSA to other relevant variables is small. Since few studies have confirmed either measure's independent validity, these measures should be used with caution until it becomes clearer what constructs they measure.

A key practice implication depends on the extent to which abilities, skills, and knowledge can be considered as elements of health literacy. While general intellectual abilities may not be readily changed, core academic skills and health-related knowledge can clearly be improved through targeted interventions. We thus suggest the use of the ASK model as an organizing framework for interventions to promote health literacy. The model not only provides for organization but also provides guidance for the assessment of intervention effects through assessment of changes in patient skills and knowledge.

Conflict of Interest

The authors state that they have no conflict of interest in the study.

Acknowledgements

This study was supported by a grant to Dr. Ownby from the US National Heart, Lung, and Blood Institute (R01HL096578). The authors also acknowledge other members of the team of investigators: Drs. Sara J. Czaja and David Loewenstein (Center on Aging at the University of Miami Miller School of Medicine), Rosemary Davenport, RN, MSN, ARNP, Study Coordinator, Dr. Ana-Maria Homs, Assessor, and Ms. Lilly Valiente who provided data management assistance.

Reference List

[1] Berkman ND, Sheridan SL, Donahue KE, Halpern DJ, Viera A, Crotty K, et al. Health literacy interventions and outcomes: an updated systematic review. Evidence report/technology assesment no. 199. Rockville, MD: Agency for Healthcare Research and Quality; 2011.

[2] Dewalt DA, Berkman ND, Sheridan S, Lohr KN, Pignone MP. Literacy and health outcomes: a systematic review of the literature. J Gen Intern Med 2004 Dec;19(12):1228-39.

[3] Berkman ND, Sheridan SL, Donahue KE, Halpern DJ, Crotty K. Low health literacy and health outcomes: an updated systematic review. Ann Intern Med 2011 Jul 19;155(2):97-107.

[4] Osborn CY, Paasche-Orlow MK, Davis TC, Wolf MS. Health literacy: An overlooked factor in understanding HIV health disparities. Am J Prev Med 2007;33(5):374-8.

[5] Osborn CY, Cavanaugh K, Wallston KA, Kripalani S, Elasy TA, Rothman RL, et al. Health literacy explains racial disparities in diabetes medication adherence. J Health Commun 2011;16 Suppl 3:268-78.

[6] Paasche-Orlow MK, Wolf MS. Promoting health literacy research to reduce health disparities. J Health Commun 2010;15 Suppl 2:34-41.

[7] Parker RM, Baker DW, Williams MV, Nurss JR. The Test of Functional Health Literacy in Adults: A new instrument for measuring patients' literacy skills. Journal of General Internal Medicine 1995;10:537-41.

[8] Murphy PW, Davis TC, Long SW, Jackson RH, Decker BC. Rapid Estimate of Adult Literacy in Medicine (REALM): A quick reading test for patients. Journal of Reading 1993;37:124-30.

[9] Lee SY, Bender DE, Ruiz RE, Cho YI. Development of an easy-to-use Spanish health literacy test. Health Serv Res 2006 Aug;41(4 Pt 1):1392-412.

[10] Pleasant A, McKinney J, Rikard RV. Health literacy measurement: a proposed research agenda. J Health Commun 2011;16 Suppl 3:11-21.

[11] Pleasant A, McKinney J. Coming to consensus on health literacy measurement: an online discussion and consensus-gauging process. Nurs Outlook 2011 Mar;59(2):95-106.

[12] Ownby RL, Waldrop-Valverde D. Health literacy is related to problem solving. Paper presented at the Health Literacy Research Conference. Washington DC: 2009.

[13] Haun J, Luther S, Dodd V, Donaldson P. Measurement variation across health literacy assessments: implications for assessment selection in research and practice. J Health Commun 2012;17 Suppl 3:141-59.

[14] Jordan JE, Osborne RH, Buchbinder R. Critical appraisal of health literacy indices revealed variable underlying constructs, narrow content and psychometric weaknesses. J Clin Epidemiol 2011 Apr;64(4):366-79.

[15] Griffin JM, Partin MR, Noorbaloochi S, Grill JP, Saha S, Snyder A, et al. Variation in estimates of limited health literacy by assessment instruments and non-response bias. J Gen Intern Med 2010 Jul;25(7):675-81.

[16] Osborn CY, Weiss BD, Davis TC, Skripkauskas S, Rodrigue C, Bass PF, et al. Measuring adult literacy in health care: performance of the newest vital sign. Am J Health Behav 2007 Sep;31 Suppl 1:S36-S46.

[17] Kutner M, Greenberg E, Jin Y, Paulsen C. The health literacy of America's adults: Results from the 2003 National Asessment of Adult

Literacy (NCES 2006-483). Washington, DC: US Department of Education, National Center for Educational Statistics; 2006.

[18] Paasche-Orlow MK, Wolf MS. The causal pathways linking health literacy to health outcomes. Am J Health Behav 2007 Sep;31 Suppl 1:S19-S26.

[19] Aguirre AC, Ebrahim N, Shea JA. Performance of the English and Spanish S-TOFHLA among publicly insured Medicaid and Medicare patients. Patient Educ Couns 2005 Mar;56(3):332-9.

[20] Mottus R, Johnson W, Murray C, Wolf MS, Starr JM, Deary IJ. Towards understanding the links between health literacy and physical health. Health Psychol 2013 Feb 25.

[21] Chin J, Morrow DG, Stine-Morrow EA, Conner-Garcia T, Graumlich JF, Murray MD. The process-knowledge model of health literacy: evidence from a componential analysis of two commonly used measures. J Health Commun 2011;16 Suppl 3:222-41.

[22] Wolf MS, Curtis LM, Wilson EA, Revell W, Waite KR, Smith SG, et al. Literacy, cognitive function, and health: Results of the LitCog study. J Gen Int Med 2012;27(10):1300-7.

[23] Baker DW, Gazmararian JA, Sudano J, Patterson M, Parker RM, Williams MV. Health literacy and performance on the Mini-Mental State Examination. Aging Ment Health 2002 Feb;6(1):22-9.

[24] Cattell RB. Theory of fluid and crystallized intelligence: A critical experiment. Journal of Educational Psychology 1963;54:1-22.

[25] Horn JL, Cattell RB. Refinement and test of the theory of fluid and crystallized general intelligences. Journal of Educational Psychology 1966;57:253-70.

[26] Carroll JB. Human cognitive abilities: A survey of factor-analytic studies. Cambridge: Cambridge University Press; 1993.

[27] Folstein MF, Folstein SE, McHugh PR. "Mini-mental state." A practical method for grading the cognitive state of patients for the clinician. J Psychiatr Res 1975;12:189-98.

[28] Levinthal BR, Morrow DG, Tu W, Wu J, Murray MD. Cognition and health literacy in patients with hypertension. J Gen Intern Med 2008 Aug;23(8):1172-6.

[29] Federman AD, Sano M, Wolf MS, Siu AL, Halm EA. Health literacy and cognitive performance in older adults. J Am Geriatr Soc 2009 Aug;57(8):1475-80.

[30] Yost KJ, DeWalt DA, Lindquist LA, Hahn EA. The association between health literacy and indicators of cognitive impairment in a diverse sample of primary care patients. Patient Educ Couns 2013 Aug 8;Published online August 8, 2013.

[31] Zarcadoolas C, Pleasant A, Greer DS. Understanding health literacy: an expanded model. Health Promotion International 2005 Jun;20(2):195-203.

[32] Nutbeam D. The evolving concept of health literacy. Soc Sci Med 2008 Dec;67(12):2072-8.

[33] Baker DW. The meaning and the measure of health literacy. J Gen Intern Med 2006 Aug;21(8):878-83.

[34] Deary IJ, Pattie A, Starr JM. The stability of intelligence from age 11 to age 90 years: The Lothian birth cohort of 1921. Psychol Sci 2013 Oct 1.

[35] Kruidenier JR, MacArthur CA, Wrigley HS. Adult education literacy instruction: A review of the research. Washington, DC: National Institute for Literacy; 2010.

[36] Sørensen K, Van den Broucke S, Fullam J, Doyle G, Pelikan J, Slonska Z, et al. Health literacy and public health: a systematic review

and integration of definitions and models. BMC Public Health 2012;12:80.

[37] Nielsen-Bohlman L, Panzer AM, Kindig DA. Health literacy: A prescription to end confusion. Washington DC: National Academies Press; 2004.

[38] Parker RM, Baker DW, Williams MV, Nurss JR. The Test of Functional Health Literacy in Adults: A new instrument for measuring patients' literacy skills. J Gen Intern Med 1995 Oct;10(10):537-41.

[39] Bass PF, III, Wilson JF, Griffith CH. A shortened instrument for literacy screening. J Gen Intern Med 2003 Dec;18(12):1036-8.

[40] Rothman RL, Malone R, Bryant B, Wolfe C, Padgett P, Dewalt DA, et al. The Spoken Knowledge in Low Literacy in Diabetes scale: a diabetes knowledge scale for vulnerable patients. Diabetes Educ 2005 Mar;31(2):215-24.

[41] Gazmararian JA, Williams MV, Peel J, Baker DW. Health literacy and knowledge of chronic disease. Patient Educ Couns 2003 Nov;51(3):267-75.

[42] Hicks G, Barragan M, Franco-Paredes C, Williams MV, Del RC. Health literacy is a predictor of HIV/AIDS knowledge. Fam Med 2006 Nov;38(10):717-23.

[43] Ownby RL, Acevedo A, Waldrop-Valverde D, Jacobs RJ, Homs AM, Czaja SJ, et al. Development and initial validation of a computer-administered health literacy assessment in Spanish and English: FLIGHT/VIDAS. Patient Related Outcome Measures 2013;4:1-15.

[44] Hauser RM, Warren JR. Socioeconomic indexes for occupations: A review, update, and critique. Madison, WI: Center for Demography and Ecology. Online at http://www.ssc.wisc.edu/cde/cdewp/96-01.pdf.; 1996.

[45] Shavers VL. Measurement of socioeconomic status in

health disparities research. J Natl Med Assoc 2007 Sep;99(9):1013-23.

[46] Adler NE, Ostrove JM. Socioeconomic status and health: What we know and what we don't. Ann NY Acad Sci 2013;896:3-15.

[47] Vyas S, Kumaranayake L. Constructing socio-economic status indices: how to use principal components analysis. Health Policy and Planning 2006 Nov 1;21(6):459-68.

[48] Woodcock RW, McGrew KS, Mather N. Woodcock-Johnson III Normative Update. Rolling Meadows, IL: Riverside; 2007.

[49] Woodcock RW, Muñoz-Sandoval AF, McGrew KS, Mather N. Batería III Woodcock-Muñoz. Rolling Meadows, IL: Riverside; 2007.

[50] Wechsler D. Manual for the Wechsler Adult Intelligence Scale--Third Edition (WAIS-III). San Antonio TX: Pearson Assessment; 1997.

[51] Brinch CN, Galloway TA. Schooling in adolescence raises IQ scores. Proc Natl Acad Sci U S A 2012 Jan 10;109(2):425-30.

[52] Baker DW, Dewalt DA, Schillinger D, Hawk V, Ruo B, Bibbins-Domingo K, et al. The effect of progressive, reinforcing telephone education and counseling versus brief educational intervention on knowledge, self-care behaviors and heart failure symptoms. J Card Fail 2011 Oct;17(10):789-96.

[53] Baker DW, Dewalt DA, Schillinger D, Hawk V, Ruo B, Bibbins-Domingo K, et al. "Teach to goal": theory and design principles of an intervention to improve heart failure self-management skills of patients with low health literacy. J Health Commun 2011;16 Suppl 3:73-88.

[54] Dewalt DA, Davis TC, Wallace AS, Seligman HK, Bryant-Shilliday B, Arnold CL, et al. Goal setting in diabetes self-management: taking the baby steps to success. Patient Educ Couns 2009 Nov;77(2):218-23.

[55] Paasche-Orlow MK, Riekert KA, Bilderback A, Chanmugam A, Hill P, Rand CS, et al. Tailored education may reduce health literacy disparities in asthma self-management. Am J Respir Crit Care Med 2005 Oct 15;172(8):980-6.

[56] Ownby RL, Waldrop-Valverde D, Caballero J, Jacobs RJ. Baseline medication adherence and response to an electronically delivered health literacy intervention targeting adherence. Neurobehav HIV Med 2012 Oct 18;4:113-21.

[57] Baker DW, Williams MV, Parker RM, Gazmararian JA, Nurss J. Development of a brief test to measure functional health literacy. Patient Educ Couns 1999 Sep;38(1):33-42.

Table 1. Sample Description

	English Mean (SD)	Spanish Mean (SD)
N	161	198
Age	52.5 (17.5)	49.8 (15.6)
Years of Education	13.6 (2.3)	12.4 (2.8)
Income	$31, 188	$27,889
SEIa	44.6 (22.4)	39.2 (20.1)
SES Factor Scoreb	0.19 (0.80)	-0.14 (0.82)
Crystallizedc	95.9 (10.6)	89.6 (9.0)
Fluidd	10.6 (2.3)	10.6 (2.7)
WJ Passage Comprehensionc	97.4 (11.0)	94.8 (11.2)
WJ Applied Problemsc	97.1 (11.30)	87.1 (10.4)
Health Knowledged	8.8 (3.1)	7.5 (2.6)
TOFHLA Readinge	46.4 (4.4)	43.3 (7.6)
TOFHLA Numeracye	47.8 (2.8)	43.5 (6.1)
	English N	Spanish N
Gender: Men/Women	70/91	81/118
Race: White/Black	91/70	198/0

aThe occupation socioeconomic index ranges from 0 to 100; bFactor score index combining education, income and socioeconomic index with mean of 0 and standard deviation of 0; cThis score has a mean of 100 and standard deviation of 15; dAverage of scaled scores that each have a mean of 10 and standard deviation of 3; dRaw score on scale with maximum of 15; eMaximum total score for each is 50.

Table 2. ASK Predictors of TOFHLA Reading Scores (Combined Sample)

	Model 1: Demographics				Model 2: Abilities			
	B	SE	t	p	B	SE	t	p
Intercept	57.80	2.69	21.51	< 0.001	28.86	4.02	7.18	< 0.001
Age	-0.09	0.02	-4.59	< 0.001	-0.07	0.02	-4.13	< 0.001
SES	1.93	0.33	5.85	< 0.001	0.97	0.30	3.23	0.001
Female Gender	0.51	0.54	0.94	0.35	1.56	0.48	3.26	0.001
Black Race	-3.10	0.86	-3.62	< 0.001	-0.93	0.77	-1.21	0.23
Spanish Language	-3.22	0.72	-4.46	< 0.001	-1.17	0.67	-1.74	0.08/
Crystallized					0.16	0.03	5.30	< 0.001
Fluid					0.56	0.11	5.06	< 0.001
Reading								
Knowledge								

Model 3: Skills				Model 4: Knowledge			
B	SE	t	p	B	SE	t	p
26.79	4.01	6.68	< 0.001	27.83	3.98	7.00	< 0.001
-0.08	0.02	-4.57	< 0.001	-0.09	0.02	-4.93	< 0.001
0.79	0.30	2.62	0.009	0.55	0.31	1.76	0.08
1.50	0.47	3.17	0.002	1.23	0.48	2.59	0.01
-0.96	0.76	-1.27	0.21	-0.72	0.75	-0.96	0.34
-1.40	0.67	-2.10	0.04	-1.23	0.66	-1.86	0.06
0.10	0.03	3.02	0.003	0.08	0.04	2.18	0.03
0.47	0.11	4.13	< 0.001	0.46	0.11	4.15	< 0.001
0.09	0.03	3.14	0.002	0.09	0.03	2.95	0.003
				0.28	0.10	2.86	0.01

Table 3. ASK Predictors of TOFHLA Numeracy Scores (Combined Sample)

	Model 1: Demographics				Model 2: Abilities			
	B	SE	t	p	B	SE	t	p
Intercept	56.31	2.89	19.48	< 0.001	43.12	4.86	8.87	< 0.001
Age	-0.04	0.02	-1.72	0.09	-0.03	0.02	-1.28	0.20
SES	0.85	0.36	2.39	0.02	0.38	0.37	1.03	0.30
Female Gender	0.39	0.58	0.68	0.50	0.92	0.58	1.58	0.12
Black Race	-1.67	0.92	-1.81	0.07	-0.61	0.94	-0.65	0.51
Spanish Language	-4.94	0.78	-6.35	< 0.001	-4.06	0.82	-4.97	< 0.001
Crystallized					0.06	0.04	1.68	0.10
Fluid					0.34	0.14	2.54	0.01
Math								
Knowledge								

Model 3: Skills				Model 4: Knowledge			
B	SE	t	p	B	SE	t	p
38.64	5.34	7.24	< 0.001	39.40	5.33	7.40	< 0.001
-0.03	0.02	-1.29	0.20	-0.03	0.02	-1.52	0.13
0.26	0.37	0.70	0.49	0.05	0.38	0.12	0.90
1.14	0.59	1.93	0.054	0.92	0.60	1.53	0.13
-0.43	0.93	-0.46	0.65	-0.24	0.94	-0.26	0.80
-3.49	0.86	-4.05	< 0.001	-3.37	0.86	-3.92	< 0.001
0.03	0.04	0.91	0.37	0.01	0.04	0.23	0.82
0.24	0.14	1.70	0.10	0.23	0.14	1.64	0.10
0.07	0.04	1.98	0.049	0.07	0.04	2.00	0.047
				0.23	0.12	1.89	0.06

Table 4. ASK Predictors of REALM scores (English Speakers Only)

	Model 1: Demographics				Model 2: Abilities			
	B	SE	t	p	B	SE	t	p
Intercept	64.32	3.37	19.11	< 0.001	43.62	6.17	7.06	< 0.001
Age	-0.01	0.03	-0.19	0.85	-0.01	0.03	-0.34	0.74
SES	1.00	0.60	1.68	0.10	0.09	0.61	0.15	0.88
Female Gender	2.38	0.96	2.46	0.02	2.86	0.93	3.09	0.002
Black Race	-3.42	1.16	-2.96	< 0.001	-2.61	1.17	-2.23	0.03
Crystallized					0.21	0.06	3.51	0.001
Fluid					-0.07	0.25	-0.26	0.80
Reading								
Knowledge								

Model 3: Skills				Model 4: Knowledge			
B	SE	t	p	B	SE	t	p
39.68	6.33	6.27	< 0.001	41.84	5.94	7.04	< 0.001
-0.02	0.03	-0.70	0.49	-0.03	0.03	-1.17	0.25
-0.26	0.62	-0.42	0.67	-0.91	0.60	-1.52	0.13
2.91	0.91	3.19	0.002	2.09	0.87	2.39	0.02
-2.65	1.15	-2.30	0.02	-1.88	1.09	-1.72	0.09
0.12	0.07	1.79	0.08	0.05	0.07	0.78	0.44
-0.20	0.26	-0.80	0.42	-0.21	0.24	-0.88	0.38
0.14	0.06	2.24	0.03	0.13	0.06	2.20	0.03
				0.79	0.18	4.45	< 0.001

Table 5. ASK Predictors of SAHLSA Scores (Spanish Speakers Only)

	Model 1: Demographicsa				Model 2: Abilities			
	B	SE	t	p	B	SE	t	p
Intercept	42.40	2.10	20.20	< 0.001	29.38	6.12	4.80	< 0.001
Age	0.01	0.04	0.19	0.85	0.04	0.04	0.91	0.36
SES	1.42	0.55	2.58	0.01	1.19	0.57	2.09	0.04
Female Gender	1.71	0.92	1.87	0.06	1.83	0.97	1.89	0.06
Crystallized					0.15	0.06	2.34	0.02
Fluid					-0.15	0.20	-0.73	0.47
Reading								
Knowledge								

aModels do not include race as all Spanish-speaking participants identified themselves as white.

Model 3: Skills				Model 4: Knowledge			
B	SE	t	p	B	SE	t	p
27.17	6.25	4.35	< 0.001	29.98	6.44	4.65	< 0.001
0.03	0.04	0.77	0.44	0.02	0.04	0.50	0.262
1.06	0.57	1.86	0.07	0.76	0.60	1.27	0.21
1.67	0.97	1.73	0.09	1.38	0.98	1.41	0.16
0.10	0.07	1.40	0.16	0.06	0.07	0.80	0.43
-0.24	0.21	-1.16	0.25	-0.24	0.21	-1.16	0.25
0.09	0.05	1.58	0.12	0.08	0.05	1.39	0.17
				0.34	0.21	1.64	0.10

Table 6. Percent of variability (R2) accounted for in regression models

	TOFHLA Reading	TOFHLA Numeracy	REALM	SAHLSA
Demographics	19	18	17	7
Abilities	22	3	5	3
Skills	2	0	3	2
Knowledge	1	1	5	2
Total	44	22	34	14

IV Tables

Normative Data

As discussed in Chapter 5, F/V users may have one or more purposes in using the scale. One key issue in interpreting a person's score on any scale is understanding their level of performance. Age-group based normative data allow an understanding of how a person's score is related to other persons of similar age. This can be contrasted with cutoff scores, which are designed to target a specific level of ability.

The tables that follow are the same as those provided in Chapter 5, reproduced at the end of this manual for easy reference. The standard scores provided are T scores. This form of standard score has an average value of 50 and a standard deviation of 10. They can be interpreted according to the following table.

Table A-1. Guide to Interpreting T scores

Range	Interpretation
Greater than 60	Above Average
40-60	Average
30-40	Below Average
Less than 30	Significantly Below Average

Table A-2. Available F/V scales

Scale	Access	Items	Time	Purpose
Paper	Paper	20	15-20	Assess general health literacy
Screen	Paper	10	10-12	Screen for low health literacy
HL40	Computer	40	20-30	Diagnostic assessment of prose and document health literacy
NUM	Computer	29	20-30	Diagnostic assessment of numeracy skills
LIS	Computer	13	15	Assess listening skills in simulated clinical encounter, patient education, and research settings
FACT	Computer	14	15	Assessment of conceptual health knowlege

Information on how to access computer scales and to obtain test materials for paper and pencil scales is available at www.flightvidas.org.

w

Table A-3. T Score Equivalents of Raw Scores on the English 20-item HL Scale

Raw Score	18-29	30-39	40-49	50-59	60-69	70 and older
1	2	14	26	18	22	22
2	5	17	28	20	25	24
3	8	19	30	23	27	26
4	11	21	32	25	29	28
5	14	24	34	27	31	30
6	17	26	36	30	33	32
7	21	28	37	32	35	34
8	24	31	39	34	37	36
9	27	33	41	37	39	39
10	30	35	43	39	41	41
11	33	38	45	42	44	43
12	36	40	47	44	46	45
13	39	42	49	46	48	47
14	42	45	51	49	50	49
15	45	47	53	51	52	51
16	48	49	55	53	54	53
17	51	52	57	56	56	55
18	54	54	58	58	58	57
19	57	56	60	60	60	59
20	60	59	62	63	63	61

Table A-4. T Score Equivalents of Raw Scores on the Spanish 20-item HL Scale

Raw Score	18-29	30-39	40-49	50-59	60-69	70 and older
1	12	13	21	27	33	35
2	15	16	23	29	35	37
3	17	18	25	31	37	40
4	20	21	28	33	39	42
5	23	23	30	35	41	44
6	25	26	32	37	43	47
7	28	28	34	39	45	49
8	31	31	36	40	47	52
9	33	33	39	42	49	54
10	36	36	41	44	51	56
11	39	38	43	46	53	59
12	41	41	45	48	55	61
13	44	43	47	50	57	64
14	46	46	50	52	59	66
15	49	48	52	54	61	68
16	52	50	54	56	63	71
17	54	53	56	58	65	73
18	57	55	58	60	67	76
19	60	58	61	62	69	78
20	62	60	63	64	71	80

Table A-5. T Score Equivalents of Raw Scores on the English 10-item Screening Tool

Raw Score	18-29	30-39	40-49	50-59	60-69	70 and older
1	10	16	30	25	26	26
2	15	21	33	29	30	29
3	21	26	37	33	34	33
4	26	30	40	37	38	37
5	32	35	44	41	42	41
6	37	39	47	45	45	45
7	43	44	51	49	49	49
8	48	49	55	52	53	52
9	53	53	58	56	57	56
10	59	58	62	60	61	60

Table A-6. T Score Equivalents of Raw Scores on the Spanish 10-item Screening Tool

Raw Score	18-29	30-39	40-49	50-59	60-69	70 and older
1	11	18	20	30	34	39
2	16	23	24	33	38	43
3	22	27	29	37	42	47
4	27	32	33	40	46	52
5	33	36	38	44	50	56
6	38	40	42	47	54	60
7	44	45	47	51	58	64
8	49	49	52	54	62	68
9	55	54	56	58	66	73
10	61	58	61	61	70	77

Printed in Dunstable, United Kingdom

91218880R00105